Mosby

A Harcourt Health Sciences Company

St. Louis   London   Philadelphia   Sydney   Toro

Kevin T. Patton
Professor of Life Science
St. Charles County Community College
St. Peters, Missouri

Adjunct Assistant Professor of Physiology
Saint Louis University Medical School
St. Louis, Missouri

Gary A. Thibodeau
Chancellor and Professor of Biology
University of Wisconsin–River Falls
River Falls, Wisconsin

Mosby's Handbook of Anatomy & Physiology

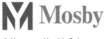

A Harcourt Health Sciences Company

Vice President, Nursing Editorial Director: *Sally Schrefer*
Executive Editor: *June Thompson*
Developmental Editor: *Billi Sharp*
Project Manager: *John Rogers*
Project Specialist: *Kathleen L. Teal*
Designer: *Kathi Gosche*

Mosby, Inc.
11830 Westline Industrial Drive
St. Louis, Missouri 63146

International Standard Book Number   0-323-01096-2

00 01 02 03 04 GW H / 9 8 7 6 5 4 3 2 1

reface

WHO NEEDS A HANDBOOK OF THE STRUCTURE AND FUNCTION OF THE HUMAN BODY? The anatomy and physiology of the human body is a wonderfully complex study. A study that forms the basis of understanding the everyday workings of our own bodies. It also forms the basis of all of the clinical and applied human sciences. But because of its complexity, we don't always remember all the little details. This is true especially if we haven't reviewed them recently—or never learned them the first place. Well, here they are! All those little bits of handy information presented in an easy-to-interpret collection of diagrams, labeled photographs, and concise tables.

For those of you in the health professions, this handbook will be a useful "mini-reference" you can carry with you as you work. It contains all of those little details that you know you know but can't seem to remember at the moment. Perhaps even more importantly, you'll have an incredibly effective tool for patient teaching always at your fingertips!

For those of you in related fields such as medical transcription, medical or liability insurance, health information technology, law, physical education and sports, recreation, law enforcement, teaching, human services, fiction and nonfiction writing and journalism, and so on, you will find this handbook to be an invaluable tool. It allows you find and understand all the basic concepts of human body structure and function so you can do your job more easily and effectively.

Even those of you who have no professional need for such a tool as this handbook will find it to be an important part of your household or office reference library. We're all humans and we all have occasion to wonder about how our body is built and how it works—especially when we are sick or think we may be. Using this handbook, you will more clearly understand what your physician is saying to you. In fact, you might want to bring this handbook along next time you visit a clinic, hospital, or professional office. And what better tool is there to help you explain the structure and function of the body to an inquisitive child?

HOW DO I USE THIS HANDBOOK? Because this is a handbook, you should keep it "at hand." When you have need for quickly finding information about human structure or function, simply grab it and thumb through its pages. The first four chapters of the handbook lay out the "basic sciences" of the human body. These include the overall "Organization of the Body" (Ch. 1), "Body Chemistry" (Ch. 2), "Cells: The Basic Units of the Body" (Ch. 3) and "Tissues: The Fabric of the Body" (Ch. 4). The remainder of the handbook is organized by body system: skin, skeletal, muscular, and so on. Either a quick glance at the Contents (p. vii) or simply flipping through the pages of the handbook should get you to where you want to be in a moment.

Once you've located the information you are looking for, use all the little features we have provided to make things clearer. *First,* there is an anatomical rosette in all figures of body parts. This rosette, like the directional compass rosette found on maps, orients you quickly to which way is "up" and which way is "down" in the body part(s) shown. We have included a handy summary of our "anatomical rosette" inside the front cover for easy reference. *Second,* nearly every figure, diagram, and photograph has a concise, helpful narrative explaining its content. *Third,* the careful use of color to show realistic structure, to highlight different areas of important diagrams, and to contrast different concepts within tables, will help you find what you are looking for quickly and easily.

This handbook is the product of many years of teaching and writing and we can't possibly mention all of the literally hundreds who have contributed to this effort in one way or another. However, we would especially like to mention the following: Developmental Editor/Writer, Gail Brower; Developmental Editor, Billi Sharp; Executive Editor, June Thompson; Vice President, Nursing Editorial Director, Sally Schrefer; Project Specialist, Kathy Teal; and Designer, Kathi Gosche. Every writing team should be so fortunate as to have a support network as talented, good-humored, hard-working, professional, and fun as we have!

Kevin Patton
Gary Thibodeau

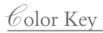

Color Key

For Select Anatomical Structures and Biochemical Compounds

Biochemistry

- Carbon
- Chloride
- Energy (ATP)
- Hydrogen
- Nitrogen
- Oxygen
- Potassium
- Sodium
- Sulfur

Other structures

- Afferent (sensory) pathway
- Artery
- Bone
- Efferent (motor) pathway
- Hormone
- Muscle
- Nerve
- Schwann cell
- Vein

Cellular structures

- Axon
- Cytosol
- Golgi apparatus
- Mitochondrion
- Na$^+$ channel
- Nucleus
- Plasma membrane

Contents

CHAPTER *8*   **NERVOUS SYSTEM,** 232

CHAPTER *13*

CHAPTER 1

Organization of the Body

Anatomy

Anatomy is often defined as the study of the structure of an organism and the relationships of its parts. The word *anatomy* is derived from two Greek words (*ana*, "apart," and *temos* or *tomos*, "cutting"). Students of anatomy still learn about the structure of the human body by literally cutting it apart. This process, called *dissection*, remains a principal technique used to isolate and study the structural components or parts of the human body.

Biology is defined as the study of life. Both anatomy and physiology are subdivisions of this very broad area of inquiry. Just as biology can be subdivided into specific areas for study, so can anatomy and physiology. For example, the term *gross anatomy* is used to describe the study of body parts visible to the naked eye. Before the discovery of the microscope, anatomists had to study human structure using only their eyes during dissection. These early anatomists could make only a *gross*, or whole, examination. With the use of modern microscopes, many anatomists now specialize in *microscopic anatomy*, including the study of cells, called *cytology* (sye-TOL-o-jee), and tissues, called *histology* (his-TOL-o-jee).

Other branches of anatomy include the study of human growth and development (*developmental anatomy*) or the study of diseased body structures (*pathological anatomy*). In this handbook, the body is presented by systems—a process called *systemic anatomy*. Systems are groups of organs that have a common function, such as the bones in the skeletal system and the muscles in the muscular system.

Physiology

Physiology is the science of the functions of the living organism and its parts. The term is a combination of two Greek words (*physis,* "nature," and *logos,* "science or study"). Simply stated, it is the study of physiology that helps us understand how the body works. Physiologists attempt to discover and understand, through active experimentation, the intricate control systems and regulatory mechanisms that permit the body to operate and survive in an often hostile environment. As a scientific discipline, physiology can be subdivided according to (1) the type of organism involved, such as human physiology or plant physiology; (2) the organizational level studied, such as molecular or cellular physiology; or (3) a specific or *systemic* function being studied, such as neurophysiology, respiratory physiology, or cardiovascular physiology.

Anatomical Position and Bilateral Symmetry

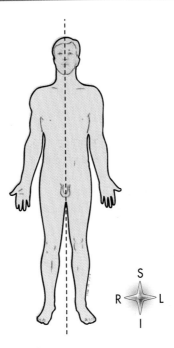

In the anatomical position, the body is in an erect, or standing, posture with the arms at the sides and palms forward. The head and feet are also pointing forward. The *dotted line* in the illustration above shows the body's bilateral symmetry. As a result of this organizational feature, the right and left sides of the body are mirror images of each other.

*B*ody Cavities

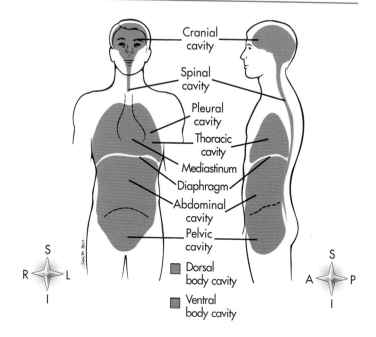

Cranial cavity

Spinal cavity

Pleural cavity

Thoracic cavity

Mediastinum

Diaphragm

Abdominal cavity

Pelvic cavity

- ▢ Dorsal body cavity
- ▢ Ventral body cavity

S
R — L
I

S
A — P
I

Location and subdivisions of the major body cavities.

Organs in Ventral Body Cavities

Areas	Organs
THORACIC CAVITY	
Right pleural cavity	Right lung (in pleural cavity)
Mediastinum	Heart (in pericardial cavity)
	Trachea
	Right and left bronchi
	Esophagus
	Thymus gland
	Aortic arch and thoracic aorta
	Venae cavae
	Various lymph nodes and nerves
	Thoracic duct
Left pleural cavity	Left lung (in pleural cavity)
ABDOMINOPELVIC CAVITY	
Abdominal cavity	Liver
	Gallbladder
	Stomach
	Pancreas
	Intestines
	Spleen
	Kidneys
	Ureters
Pelvic cavity	Urinary bladder
	Female reproductive organs
	Uterus
	Uterine tubes
	Ovaries
	Male reproductive organs
	Prostate gland
	Seminal vesicles
	Parts of vas deferens
	Part of large intestine, namely, sigmoid colon and rectum

Specific Body Regions

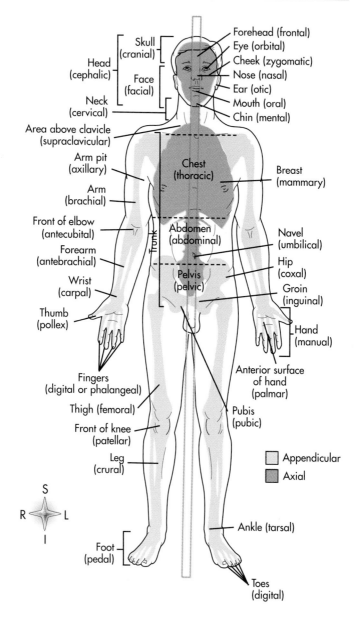

Head (cephalic)
- Skull (cranial)
- Face (facial)

Neck (cervical)

Forehead (frontal)
Eye (orbital)
Cheek (zygomatic)
Nose (nasal)
Ear (otic)
Mouth (oral)
Chin (mental)

Area above clavicle (supraclavicular)
Arm pit (axillary)
Arm (brachial)
Front of elbow (antecubital)
Forearm (antebrachial)
Wrist (carpal)
Thumb (pollex)

Chest (thoracic)
Trunk
Abdomen (abdominal)
Pelvis (pelvic)

Breast (mammary)
Navel (umbilical)
Hip (coxal)
Groin (inguinal)
Hand (manual)
Anterior surface of hand (palmar)

Fingers (digital or phalangeal)
Thigh (femoral)
Front of knee (patellar)
Leg (crural)

Pubis (pubic)

Appendicular
Axial

S
R — L
I

Ankle (tarsal)

Foot (pedal)

Toes (digital)

Note that the body as a whole can be subdivided into two major portions or components: axial and appendicular.

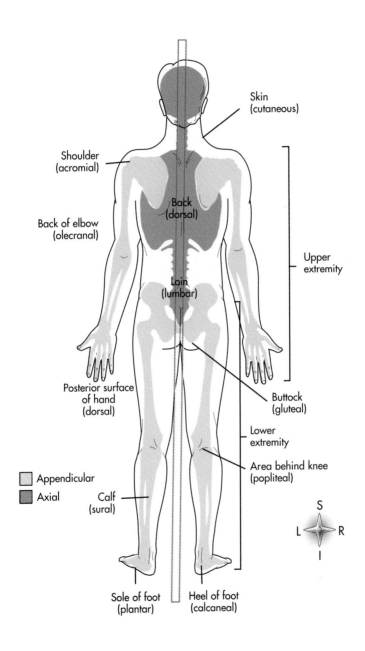

Skin
(cutaneous)

Shoulder
(acromial)

Back
(dorsal)

Back of elbow
(olecranal)

Loin
(lumbar)

Upper
extremity

Posterior surface
of hand
(dorsal)

Buttock
(gluteal)

Lower
extremity

Area behind knee
(popliteal)

Appendicular
Axial

Calf
(sural)

Sole of foot
(plantar)

Heel of foot
(calcaneal)

S

L — R

I

Descriptive Terms for Body Regions

Body Region	Area or Example
Abdominal (ab-DOM-in-al)	Anterior torso below diaphragm
Acromial (ah-KRO-me-al)	Shoulder
Antebrachial (an-tee-BRAY-kee-al)	Forearm
Antecubital (an-tee-KYOO-bi-tal)	Depressed area just in front of elbow
Axillary (AK-si-lair-ee)	Armpit
Brachial (BRAY-kee-al)	Upper arm
Calcaneal (cal-CANE-ee-al)	Heel of foot
Carpal (KAR-pal)	Wrist
Cephalic (se-FAL-ik)	Head
Cervical (SER-vi-kal)	Neck
Coxal (COX-al)	Hip
Cranial (KRAY-nee-al)	Skull
Crural (KROOR-al)	Leg
Cubital (KYOO-bi-tal)	Elbow
Cutaneous (kyoo-TANE-ee-us)	Skin (or body surface)
Digital (DIJ-i-tal)	Fingers or toes
Dorsal (DOR-sal)	Back or top
Facial (FAY-shal)	Face
Buccal (BUK-al)	Cheek (inside)
Frontal (FRON-tal)	Forehead
Nasal (NAY-zal)	Nose
Oral (OR-al)	Mouth
Orbital or **ophthalmic** (OR-bi-tal or op-THAL-mik)	Eyes
Otic (O-tick)	Ear
Femoral (FEM-or-al)	Thigh
Gluteal (GLOO-tee-al)	Buttock
Inguinal (ING-gwi-nal)	Groin
Lumbar (LUM-bar)	Lower back between ribs and pelvis
Mammary (MAM-er-ee)	Breast
Manual (MAN-yoo-al)	Hand
Mental (MEN-tal)	Chin
Navel (NAY-val)	Area around navel, or umbilicus
Occipital (ok-SIP-i-tal)	Back of lower skull
Olecranal (o-LECK-ra-nal)	Back of elbow
Palmar (PAHL-mar)	Palm of hand
Patellar (pa-TELL-er)	Front of knee
Pedal (PED-al)	Foot
Pelvic (PEL-vik)	Lower portion of torso
Perineal (pair-i-NEE-al)	Area (perineum) between anus and genitals
Plantar (PLAN-tar)	Sole of foot
Pollex (POL-ex)	Thumb

Body Region	Area or Example
Popliteal (pop-li-TEE-al)	Area behind knee
Pubic (PYOO-bik)	Pubis
Supraclavicular (soo-pra-cla-VIK-yoo-lar)	Area above clavicle
Sural (SUR-al)	Calf
Tarsal (TAR-sal)	Ankle
Temporal (TEM-por-al)	Side of skull
Thoracic (tho-RAS-ik)	Chest
Zygomatic (zye-go-MAT-ik)	Cheek

Nine Regions of the Abdominopelvic Cavity

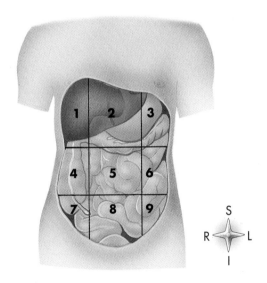

The diagram shows the most superficial organs in the abdomino-pelvic cavity.

1 Right hypochondriac region	2 Epigastric region	3 Left hypochondriac region
4 Right lumbar region	5 Umbilical region	6 Left lumbar region
7 Right iliac region	8 Hypogastric region	9 Left iliac region

Division of the Abdomen Into Four Quadrants

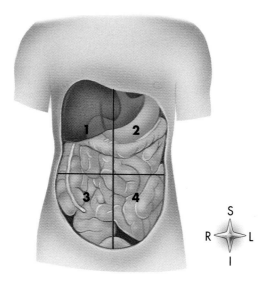

The diagram shows the relationship of internal organs to the four abdominopelvic quadrants.

1 Right upper quadrant (RUQ)	2 Left upper quadrant (LUQ)
3 Right lower quadrant (RLQ)	4 Left lower quadrant (LLQ)

Directions and Planes of the Body

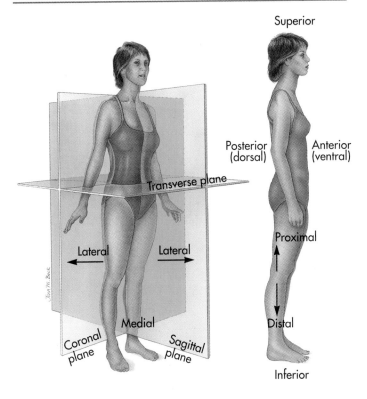

Sagittal: A lengthwise plane running from front to back is called a *sagittal* plane. Such a plane divides the body or any of its parts into right and left sides. If a sagittal section is made in the exact midline, resulting in equal and symmetrical right and left halves, the plane is called a *midsagittal* plane.

Coronal: A lengthwise plane running from side to side; divides the body or any of its parts into anterior and posterior portions; also called a *frontal* plane.

Transverse: A crosswise plane; divides the body or any of its parts into upper and lower parts; also called a *horizontal* plane.

To make the reading of anatomical figures a little easier, an *anatomical rosette* is used throughout this handbook. On many figures, you will notice a small compass rosette similar to those on geographical maps. Rather than being labeled N, S, E, and W, the anatomical rosette is labeled with abbreviated anatomical directions:

A, Anterior
D, Distal
I, Inferior
L (opposite M), Lateral
L (opposite R), Left
M, Medial
P (opposite A), Posterior
P (opposite D), Proximal
R, Right
S, Superior

$\mathscr{B}$asic Components of Homeostatic Control Mechanisms

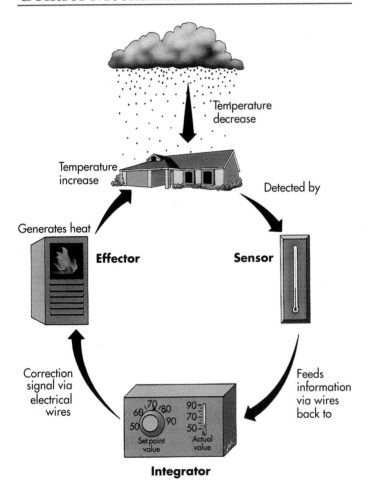

This illustration of heat from a furnace being controlled by a thermostat is a good analogy of the kind of feedback control mechanism that is also found in the human body.

$\mathcal{B}$asic Components of Homeostatic Control Mechanisms in the Body

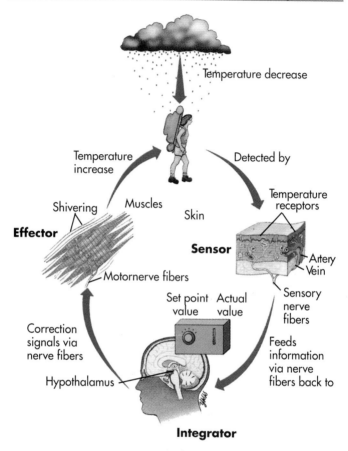

This illustrates the body's mechanism for maintaining homeostasis of body temperature. Note that in both this illustration and the one above, a stimulus (drop in temperature) activates a sensor mechanism (thermostat or body temperature receptor) that sends input to an integrating, or control, center (on-off switch or hypothalamus), which then sends input to an effector mechanism (furnace or contracting muscle). The resulting heat that is produced maintains the temperature in a "normal range." Feedback of effector activity to the sensor mechanism completes the control loop.

*M*etric Measurements and Their Equivalents

UNITS OF MEASUREMENT

Basic Unit	Metric	English	English/Metric
Time	second	second	same
Length	meter (m)	yard	1.09 yards/ 1 meter
Volume	liter (l or L)	quart	1.06 quarts/ 1 liter
Mass	gram (g)	ounce	.035 ounce/ 1 gram
Temperature	degree Celsius (°C)	degree Fahrenheit (°F)	1.8 °F/1 °C

PREFIXES

	Less Than One Basic Unit	
nano–	one billionth	.000000001
micro–	one millionth	.000001
milli–	one thousandth	.001
centi–	one hundredth	.01
deci–	one tenth	.1
	More Than One Basic Unit	
deka–	ten	10.00
hecto–	one hundred	100.00
kilo–	one thousand	1000.00
mega–	one million	1000000.00

COMMON CONVERSIONS

Multiply	By	To Get
Time		
seconds	1000	milliseconds
seconds	.00167	minutes
minutes	60	seconds
milliseconds	.001	seconds
Length		
meters	1.09	yards
meters	3.28	feet
meters	100	centimeters
meters	1000	millimeters
centimeters	.01	meters
centimeters	10	millimeters
centimeters	100000	micrometers
millimeters	.001	meters
millimeters	.1	centimeters
Volume		
liters	1.06	quarts
liters	.26	gallons
liters	1000	milliliters
liters	100	centiliters
liters	10	deciliters
centiliters	.01	liters
centiliters	10	milliliters
centiliters	.1	deciliters
deciliters	.1	liters
deciliters	10	centiliters
Mass		
grams	0.35	ounces
grams	.001	kilograms
grams	1000	milligrams
milligrams	.001	grams
kilograms	1000	grams
kilograms	2.21	pounds

As you can see from the Units of Measurement table, one "degree" in Celsius is a larger unit than one degree in Fahrenheit. In fact, a Celsius degree is 9/5 (1.8) times the size of a Fahrenheit degree. When you convert temperature readings from one form to another, this discrepancy in size must be taken into account. The 32° is added in the conversion to Fahrenheit to account for the fact that, in the Fahrenheit scale, the freezing point of water is 32°, not 0°, as it is in Celsius.

TEMPERATURE CONVERSIONS

TO CONVERT °C TO °F
Multiply °C by $\frac{9}{5}$ and add 32

____ °C $\times \frac{9}{5}$ + 32 = ____ °F

For example, to convert 35°C to °F:

35° C $\times \frac{9}{5}$ + 32 = 95° F

TO CONVERT °F TO °C
Subtract 32 from °F and multiply by $\frac{5}{9}$

(____ °F − 32) $\times \frac{5}{9}$ = ____ °C

For example, to convert 101° F to °C:

(101° F − 32) $\times \frac{5}{9}$ = 38.3° C

Body Temperatures in °Celsius and °Fahrenheit

°C	°F	°C	°F
35.0	95.0	37.8	100.0
35.1	95.2	37.9	100.2
35.2	95.4	38.0	100.4
35.3	95.6	38.1	100.6
35.4	95.8	38.2	100.8
35.5	96.0	38.3	101.0
35.7	96.2	38.4	101.2
35.8	96.4	38.6	101.4
35.9	96.6	38.7	101.6
36.0	96.8	38.8	101.8
36.1	97.0	38.9	102.0
36.2	97.2	39.0	102.2
36.3	97.4	39.1	102.4
36.4	97.6	39.2	102.6
36.6	97.8	39.3	102.8
36.7	98.0	39.4	103.0
36.8	98.2	39.6	103.2
36.9	98.4	39.7	103.4
37.0	98.6	39.8	103.6
37.1	98.8	39.9	103.8
37.2	99.0	40.0	104.0
37.3	99.2	40.1	104.2
37.4	99.4	40.2	104.4
37.6	99.6	40.3	104.6
37.7	99.8	40.4	104.8

CHAPTER 2

Body Chemistry

Biochemistry is the specialized area of chemistry that deals with living organisms and life processes. It deals directly with the chemical composition of living matter and the processes that underlie such life activities as growth, muscle contraction, and transmission of nervous impulses. An understanding of homeostatic processes and control mechanisms is in many cases dependent on knowledge of basic chemistry and on selected facts and concepts in the specialized area of biochemistry.

Periodic Table of Elements

1	2											13	14	15	16	17	18
1 H 1.008																	2 He 4.002
3 Li 6.941	4 Be 9.012											5 B 10.811	6 C 12.011	7 N 14.007	8 O 15.999	9 F 18.998	10 Ne 20.180
11 Na 22.990	12 Mg 24.305											13 Al 26.982	14 Si 28.086	15 P 30.974	16 S 32.066	17 Cl 35.452	18 Ar 39.948
19 K 39.098	20 Ca 40.078	21 Sc 44.956	22 Ti 47.867	23 V 50.942	24 Cr 51.996	25 Mn 54.931	26 Fe 55.845	27 Co 58.933	28 Ni 58.963	29 Cu 63.546	30 Zn 65.39	31 Ga 69.723	32 Ge 72.61	33 As 74.922	34 Se 78.96	35 Br 79.904	36 Kr 83.80
37 Rb 85.468	38 Sr 87.62	39 Y 88.906	40 Zr 91.224	41 Nb 92.906	42 Mo 95.94	43 Tc (98)	44 Ru 101.07	45 Rh 102.906	46 Pd 106.42	47 Ag 107.868	48 Cd 112.411	49 In 114.818	50 Sn 118.710	51 Sb 121.760	52 Te 127.60	53 I 126.904	54 Xe 131.29
55 Cs 132.905	56 Ba 137.327	57 La 138.905	72 Hf 178.49	73 Ta 180.948	74 W 183.84	75 Re 186.207	76 Os 190.23	77 Ir 192.217	78 Pt 195.08	79 Au 196.967	80 Hg 200.59	81 Tl 204.383	82 Pb 207.2	83 Bi 208.980	84 Po (209)	85 At (210)	86 Rn (222)
87 Fr (223)	88 Ra 226.025	89 Ac 227.028	104 Unq (261)	105 Unp (262)	106 Unh (263)	107 Uns (262)	108 Uno (265)	109 Une (266)	110 Uun (269)								

58 Ce 140.115	59 Pr 140.907	60 Nd 144.24	61 Pm (145)	62 Sm 150.36	63 Eu 151.965	64 Gd 157.25	65 Tb 158.925	66 Dy 162.50	67 Ho 164.930	68 Er 167.26	69 Tm 168.939	70 Yb 173.04	71 Lu 174.967
90 Th 232.038	91 Pa 231.036	92 U 238.029	93 Np 237.048	94 Pu (244)	95 Am (243)	96 Cm (247)	97 Bk (247)	98 Cf (251)	99 Es (252)	100 Fm (257)	101 Md (258)	102 No (259)	103 Lr (260)

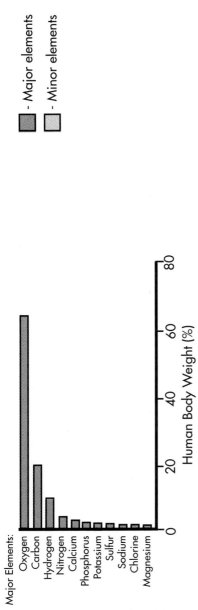

In this representation the major elements found in the body and the trace elements found in the body are distinguished by color.

Elements in the Human Body

Element	Symbol	Human Body Weight (%)	Importance or Function
MAJOR ELEMENTS			
Oxygen	O	65.0	Necessary for cellular respiration; component of water
Carbon	C	18.5	Backbone of organic molecules
Hydrogen	H	9.5	Component of water and most organic molecules; necessary for energy transfer and respiration
Nitrogen	N	3.3	Component of all proteins and nucleic acids
Calcium	Ca	1.5	Component of bones and teeth; triggers muscle contraction
Phosphorus	P	1.0	Principal component in backbone of nucleic acids; important in energy transfer
Potassium	K	0.4	Principal positive ion within cells; important in nerve function
Sulfur	S	0.3	Component of most proteins
Sodium	Na	0.2	Important positive ion surrounding cells; important in nerve function
Chlorine	Cl	0.2	Important negative ion surrounding cells
Magnesium	Mg	0.1	Component of many energy-transferring enzymes

Element	Symbol	Human Body Weight (%)	Importance or Function
TRACE ELEMENTS			
Silicone	Si	<0.1	—
Aluminum	Al	<0.1	—
Iron	Fe	<0.1	Critical component of hemoglobin in the blood
Manganese	Mn	<0.1	—
Fluorine	F	<0.1	—
Vanadium	V	<0.1	—
Chromium	Cr	<0.1	—
Copper	Cu	<0.1	Key component of many enzymes
Boron	B	<0.1	—
Cobalt	Co	<0.1	—
Zinc	An	<0.1	Key component of some enzymes
Selenium	Se	<0.1	—
Molybdenum	Mo	<0.1	Key component of many enzymes
Tin	Sn	<0.1	—
Iodine	I	<0.1	Component of thyroid hormone

$\mathcal{I}$norganic Salts Important in Body Functions

Inorganic Salt	Chemical Formula	Electrolytes
Sodium chloride	$NaCl$	$Na^+ + Cl^-$
Calcium chloride	$CaCl_2$	$Ca^{++} + 2Cl^-$
Magnesium chloride	$MgCl_2$	$Mg^{++} + 2Cl^-$
Sodium bicarbonate	$NaHCO_3$	$Na^+ + HCO_3^-$
Potassium chloride	KCl	$K^+ + Cl^-$
Sodium sulfate	Na_2SO_4	$2\,Na^+ + SO_4^=$
Calcium carbonate	$CaCO_3$	$Ca^{++} + CO_3^=$
Calcium phosphate	$Ca_3(PO_4)_2$	$3\,Ca^{++} + 2PO_4^=$

Macromolecules

Macromolecule	Subunit	Function	Example
CARBOHYDRATES			
Glycogen	Glucose	Stores energy	Liver glycogen
Ribose	Simple sugar (pentose)	Important in expression of hereditary information	Component of RNA
LIPIDS			
Triglycerides	Glycerol + 3 fatty acids	Store energy	Body fat
Phospholipids	Glycerol + 2 fatty acids + phosphate	Make up cell membranes	Plasma membrane of cell
Steroids	Steroid nucleus (4-carbon ring)	Make up cell membranes	Cholesterol
		Hormone synthesis	Estrogen
Prostaglandins	20 carbon unsaturated fatty acid containing 5-carbon ring	Regulate hormone action; enhance immune system; affect inflammatory response	Various prostaglandins
PROTEINS			
Functional	Amino acids	Regulate chemical reactions (enzymes)	Hemoglobin/Antibodies
Structural	Amino acids	Component of body support tissues	Muscle tissue
NUCLEIC ACIDS			
DNA	Nucleotides	Helps code hereditary information	Chromosomes
RNA	Nucleotides	Helps decode hereditary information	Messenger RNA

Major Functions of Human Protein Compounds

Function	Example
Provide structure	Structural proteins include keratin of skin, hair, and nails; parts of cell membranes; tendons
Catalyze chemical reactions	Lactase (enzyme in intestinal digestive juice) catalyzes chemical reaction that changes lactose to glucose and galactose
Transport substances in blood	Proteins classified as albumins combine with fatty acids to transport them in form of lipoproteins
Communicate information to cells	Insulin, a protein hormone, serves as chemical message from islet cells of the pancreas to cells all over the body
Act as receptors	Binding sites of certain proteins on surfaces of cell membranes serve as receptors for insulin and various other hormones
Defend body against many harmful agents	Proteins called *antibodies* or *immunoglobulins* combine with various harmful agents to render them harmless
Provide energy	Proteins can be metabolized for energy

Basic Structural Formula for an Amino Acid

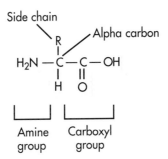

Amino acids are the basic building blocks of polypeptides, or proteins. Note the relationship in the illustration above of the side chain *(R)*, amine group, and carboxyl group to the alpha carbon. The chemical "backbone" common to all proteins is highlighted in yellow.

*F*ormation (Synthesis) and Decomposition (Hydrolysis) of a Polypeptide

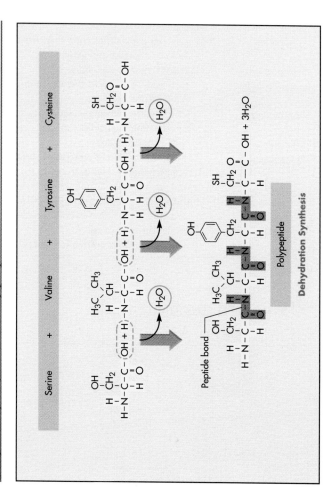

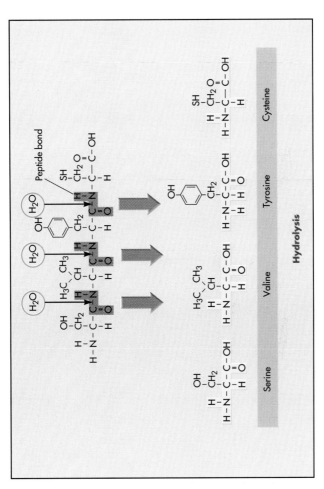

B

Part A of the illustration on pp. 26–27 shows linkage of four amino acids by three peptide bonds, resulting in the synthesis of a polypeptide chain and three molecules of water. *Part B* shows decomposition (hydrolysis) reaction, resulting from the addition of three molecules of water. Peptide bonds are broken, and individual amino acids are released.

Structural Levels of Protein

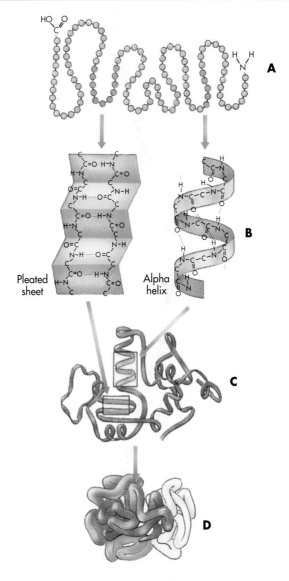

A, *Primary structure:* determined by number, kind, and sequence of amino acids in the chain. **B,** *Secondary structure:* hydrogen bonds stabilize folds or helical spirals. **C,** *Tertiary structure:* globular shape maintained by strong (covalent) intramolecular bonding and by stabilizing hydrogen bonds. **D,** *Quaternary structure:* results from bonding between more than one polypeptide unit.

*M*ajor Functions of Human Lipid Compounds

Function	Example
Energy	Lipids can be stored and broken down later for energy; they yield more energy per unit of weight than carbohydrates or proteins
Structure	Phospholipids and cholesterol are required components of cell membranes
Vitamins	Fat-soluble vitamins: vitamin A forms retinal (necessary for night vision); vitamin D increases calcium uptake; vitamin E promotes wound healing; and vitamin K is required for the synthesis of blood clotting proteins
Protection	Fat surrounds and protects organs
Insulation	Fat under the skin minimizes heat loss; fatty tissue (myelin) covers nerve cells and electrically insulates them
Regulation	Steroid hormones regulate many physiological processes. Examples: estrogen and testosterone are responsible for many of the differences between females and males; prostaglandins help regulate inflammation and tissue repair

Triglycerides

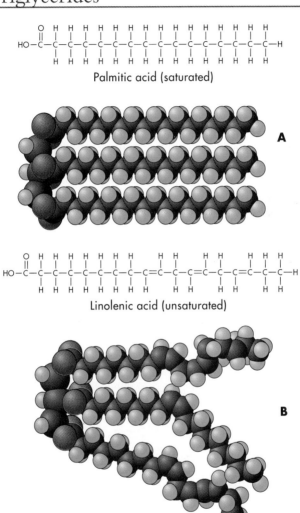

Palmitic acid (saturated)

A

Linolenic acid (unsaturated)

B

Part **A** of the three-dimensional model above shows three molecules of palmitic acid (a saturated fatty acid) joined to a molecule of glycerol, forming a triglyceride. Part **B** shows the triglyceride exhibiting "kinks" caused by the presence of double bonds in the component unsaturated fatty acids (linolenic acid).

$\mathscr{B}$lood Lipoproteins

A lipid such as cholesterol can travel in the blood only after it has attached to a protein molecule forming a lipoprotein. Some of these molecules are called *high-density lipoproteins (HDLs)* because they have a high density of protein (more protein than lipid). Another type of molecule contains less protein (and more lipid), so it is called *low-density lipoprotein (LDL)*. The composite nature of a lipoprotein molecule is shown in the illustration below.

The cholesterol in LDLs is often called "bad" cholesterol because high blood levels of LDL are associated with atherosclerosis, a life-threatening blockage of arteries. LDLs carry cholesterol *to cells,* including the cells that line blood vessels. HDLs, on the other hand, carry so-called "good" cholesterol *away from cells* and toward the liver for elimination from the body. A high proportion of HDL in the blood is associated with a low risk of developing atherosclerosis. Factors such as exercise increase HDL levels and thus decrease the risk of atherosclerosis.

The 1985 Nobel Prize in Physiology or Medicine was awarded to Drs. Michael Brown and Joseph Goldstein for their research on specialized receptor sites on LDL molecules, which are elevated in the blood of individuals with certain types of heart disease.

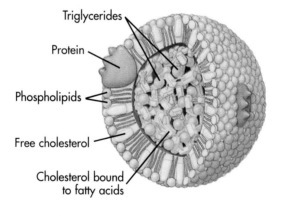

This illustrates the structure of a lipoprotein.

Phospholipid Molecules

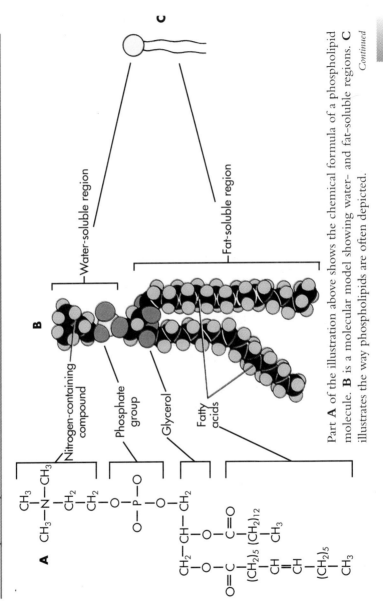

A

CH₃—N⁺—CH₃ ... (Nitrogen-containing compound)

Phosphate group

Glycerol

Fatty acids

Water-soluble region

Fat-soluble region

B

C

Part **A** of the illustration above shows the chemical formula of a phospholipid molecule. **B** is a molecular model showing water- and fat-soluble regions. **C** illustrates the way phospholipids are often depicted.

Continued

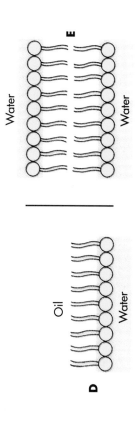

D shows the orientation of phospholipid molecules in an oil–water interface. **E** shows the orientation of phospholipid molecules when surrounded by water.

The Steroid Nucleus

A Cholesterol

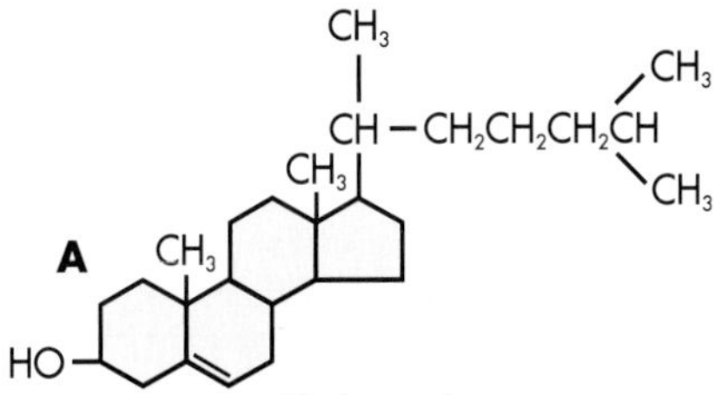

B Cortisol

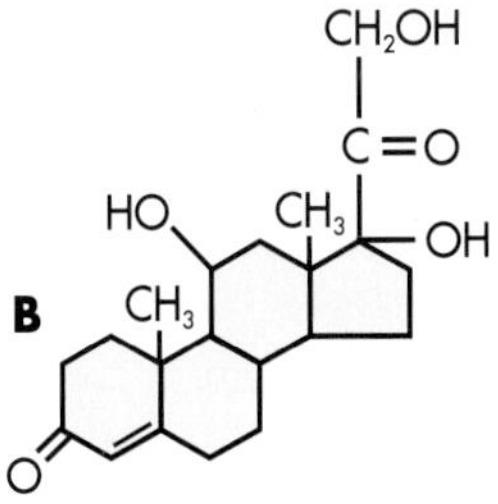

C Estrogen (estradiol)

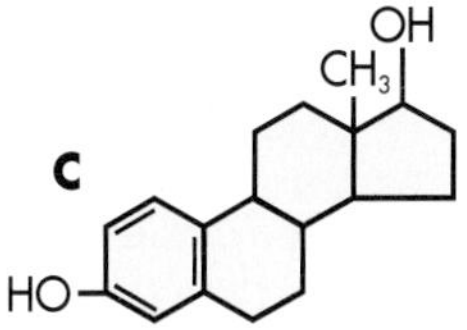

D Testosterone

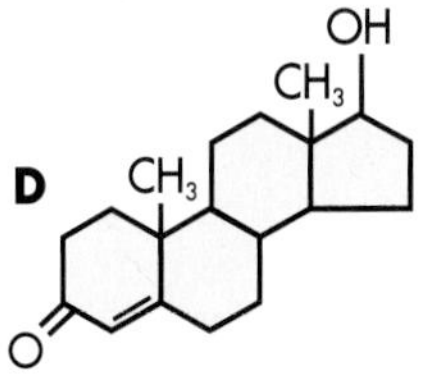

The steroid nucleus—highlighted in yellow—found in cholesterol **(A)** forms the basis for many other important compounds such as the hormones cortisol **(B)**, estradiol (an estrogen) **(C)**, and testosterone **(D)**.

Comparison of DNA and RNA Structure

	DNA	RNA
Polynucleotide strands	2	1
Sugar	Deoxyribose	Ribose
Base pairs	Adenine-thymine	Adenine-uracil
	Guanine-cytosine	Guanine-cytosine

The DNA Molecule

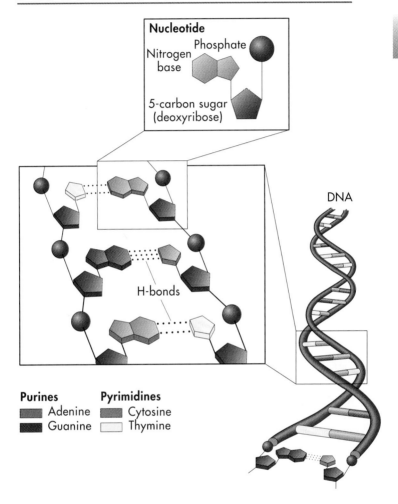

Nucleotide

Phosphate

Nitrogen base

5-carbon sugar (deoxyribose)

H-bonds

DNA

Purines
- Adenine
- Guanine

Pyrimidines
- Cytosine
- Thymine

The above representation of a DNA double helix shows the general structure of a nucleotide and the two kinds of "base pairs": adenine *(blue)* with thymine *(yellow)* and guanine *(purple)* with cytosine *(pink)*. Note that the guanine-cytosine base pair has three hydrogen bonds and the adenine-thymine base pair has two. Hydrogen bonds are extremely important in maintaining the structure of this molecule.

Adenosine Triphosphate (ATP)

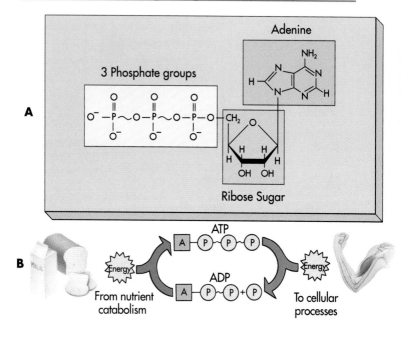

Part **A** of the above illustration shows the structure of adenosine triphosphate (ATP). A single adenosine group has three attached phosphate groups. High-energy bonds between the phosphate groups can release chemical energy to do cellular work. Part **B** shows the general scheme of the ATP energy cycle. ATP stores energy in its last high-energy phosphate bond. When that bond is later broken, energy is transferred as important intermediate compounds are formed. The adenosine diphosphate (ADP) and phosphate groups that result can be resynthesized into ATP, capturing additional energy from nutrient catabolism. Note that energy is transferred from nutrient catabolism to ADP, thus converting it to ATP, and energy is transferred *from* ATP to provide the energy required for the anabolic reactions of cellular processes as it reverts back to AD and phosphate.

3

Cells: The Basic Units of the Body

The cell theory states simply that the cell is the fundamental organizational unit of life; all living things are composed of cells. Some 100 trillion of them make up the human body.

*T*ypical (or Composite) Cell

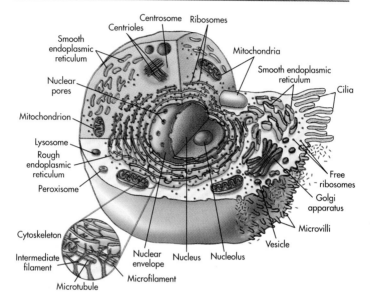

The artist's interpretation of cell structure (see above) shows the many mitochondria, known as the "power plants of the cell." Note, too, the innumerable dots bordering the endoplasmic reticulum. These are ribosomes, the cell's "protein factories."

*S*ome Major Cell Structures and Their Functions

Cell Structure	Functions
MEMBRANOUS	
Plasma membrane	Serves as the boundary of the cell, maintaining its integrity; protein molecules embedded in plasma membrane perform various functions; for example, they serve as markers that identify cells of each individual, as receptor molecules for certain hormones and other molecules, and as transport mechanisms
Endoplasmic reticulum (ER)	Ribosomes attached to rough ER synthesize proteins that leave cells via the Golgi complex; smooth ET synthesizes lipids incorporated in cell membranes, steroid hormones, and certain carbohydrates used for form glycoproteins
Golgi apparatus	Synthesizes carbohydrate, combines it with protein, and packages the product as globules of glycoprotein
Lysosomes	A cell's "digestive system"
Peroxisomes	Contain enzymes that detoxify harmful substances
Mitochondria	Catabolism; ATP synthesis; a cell's "power plants"
Nucleus	Houses the genetic code, which in turn dictates protein synthesis, thereby playing an essential role in other cell activities, namely, cell transport, metabolism, and growth
NONMEMBRANOUS	
Ribosomes	Site of protein synthesis; a cell's "protein factories"
Cytoskeleton	Acts as a framework to support the cell and its organelles; functions in cell movement; forms cell extension (microvilli, cilia, flagella)
Nucleolus	Plays an essential role in the formation of ribosomes

$\mathscr{P}$lasma Membrane

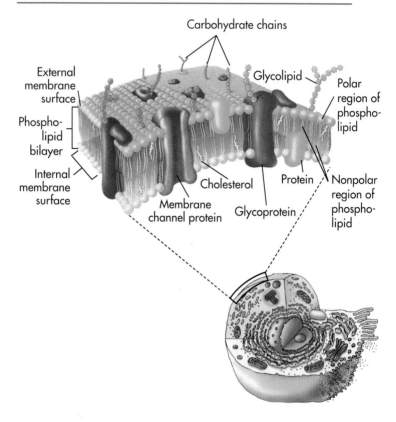

The plasma membrane is made of a bilayer of phospholipid molecules arranged with their nonpolar "tails" pointing toward each other. Cholesterol molecules help stabilize the flexible bilayer structure to prevent breakage. Protein molecules and protein-hybrid molecules may be found on the outer of inner surface of the bilayer—or, more likely, extending all the way through the membrane.

Functional Anatomy of Cell Membranes

Structure		Function
Sheet (bilayer) of phospholipids stabilized by cholesterol	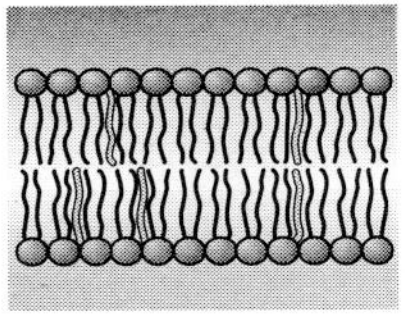	Maintain wholeness (integrity) of a cell or membranous organelle
Membrane protein that act as channels or carriers of molecules	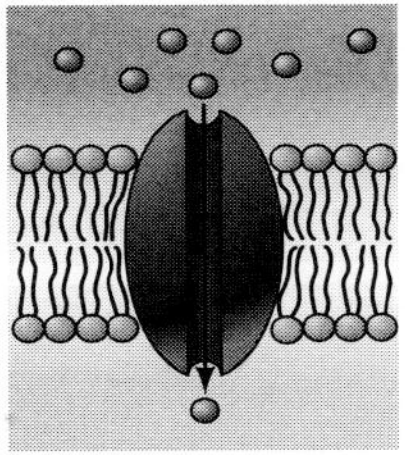	Controlled transport of water-soluble molecules from one compartment to another
Receptor molecules that trigger metabolic changes in membrane (or on other side of membrane)	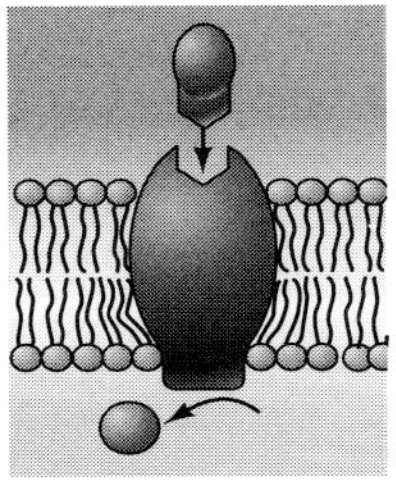	Sensitivity to hormones and other regulatory chemicals; involved in signal transduction

Continued

*F*unctional Anatomy of Cell Membranes—cont'd

Structure		Function
Enzyme molecules that catalyze specific chemical reactions	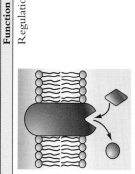	Regulation of metabolic reactions
Membrane proteins that bind to molecules outside the cell	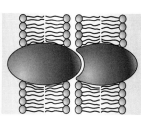	Form connections between cells and other structures such as tissue fibers or other cells

Support and maintain the shape of a cell or membranous organelle; cell movement

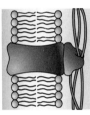

Membrane proteins that bind to support filaments within the cytoplasm

Recognition of cells or organelles

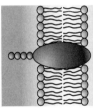

Glycoproteins or proteins in the membrane that act as markers

*F*unction of the Golgi Apparatus

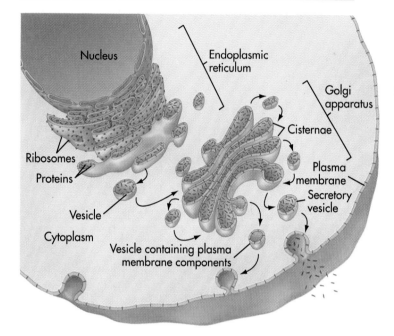

The Golgi apparatus processes and packages protein molecules delivered from the endoplasmic reticulum by small vesicles. After entering the first cisterna of the Golgi apparatus, a protein molecule undergoes a series of chemical modifications, is sent (by means of a vesicle) to the next cisterna for further modification, and so on, until it is ready to exit the last cisterna. When it is ready to exit, a molecule is packaged in a membranous secretory vesicle that migrates to the surface of the cell and "pops open" to release its contents into the space outside the cell. Some vesicles remain inside the cell for some time, serving as storage vessels for the substance to be secreted.

*M*itochondrion

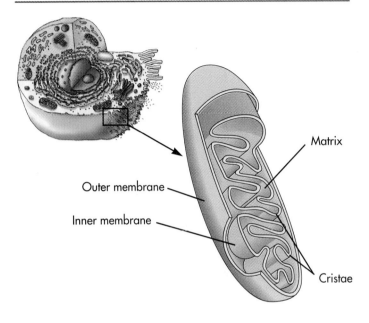

Matrix

Outer membrane

Inner membrane

Cristae

The cutaway sketch above shows outer and inner membranes. Note the many folds (cristae) of the inner membrane.

The Cytoskeleton

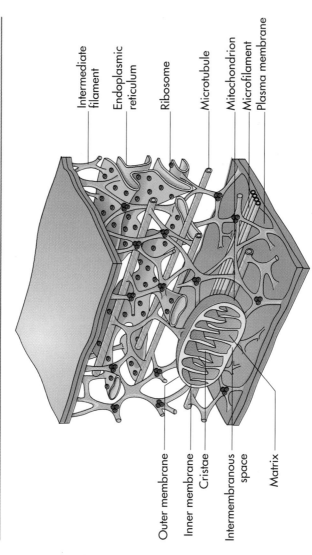

Intermediate filament
Endoplasmic reticulum
Ribosome
Microtubule
Mitochondrion
Microfilament
Plasma membrane

Outer membrane
Inner membrane
Cristae
Intermembranous space
Matrix

The artist's interpretation above shows the cell's internal framework. Notice that the "free" ribosomes and other organelles are not really free at all. Detailed structure of the mitochondrion is also labeled.

Cell Connections

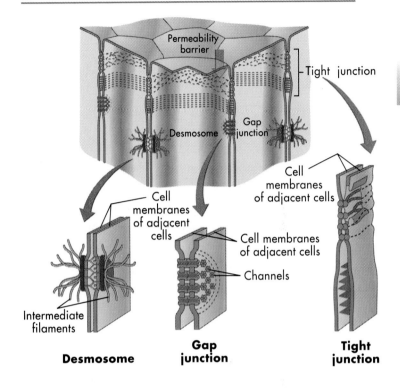

The major types of direct cell connections are desmosome, gap junction, and tight junction.

*S*ome Important Transport Processes

Process	Type	Description		Examples
Simple diffusion	Passive	Movement of particles through the phospholipid bilayer or through channels from an area of high concentration to an area of low concentration—that is, down the concentration gradient		Movement of carbon dioxide out of all cells; movement of sodium ions into nerve cells as they conduct an impulse
Dialysis	Passive	Diffusion of small solute particles, but not larger solute particles, through a selectively permeable membrane; results in separation of large and small solutes		During procedure called *peritoneal dialysis*, small solutes diffuse from blood vessels but blood proteins do not (thus removing only small solutes from the blood)
Osmosis	Passive	Diffusion of water through a selectively permeable membrane in the presence of at least one impermeant solute		Diffusion of water molecules into and out of cells to correct imbalances in water concentration

Continued

Facilitated diffusion	Passive	Diffusion of particles through a membrane by means of carrier molecules; also called *carrier-mediated passive transport*	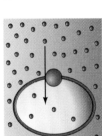	Movement of glucose molecules into most cells
Active transport	Active	Movement of solute particles from an area of low concentration to an area of high concentration (up the concentration gradient) by means of a carrier molecule	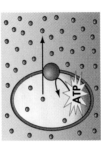	In muscle cells, pumping of nearly all calcium ions to special compartments—or out of the cell
Phagocytosis	Active	Movement of cells or other large particles into cell by trapping it in a section of plasma membrane that pinches off to form an intracellular vesicle; type of *endocytosis*	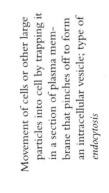	Trapping of bacterial cells by phagocytic white blood cells

*S*ome Important Transport Processes—cont'd

Process	Type	Description		Examples
Pinocytosis	Active	Movement of fluid and dissolved molecules into a cell by trapping them in a section of plasma membrane that pinches off to form an intracellular vesicle; type of *endocytosis*		Trapping of large protein molecules by some body cells
Exocytosis	Active	Movement of proteins or other cell products out of the cell by fusing a secretory vesicle with the plasma membrane		Secretion of the hormone, prolactin, by pituitary cells

$\mathcal{M}$embrane Channels

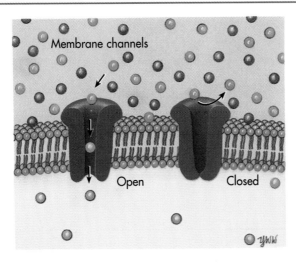

Gated channel proteins form tunnels through which specific molecules may pass—as long as the "gates" are open. Notice in the illustration above that the transported molecules move from an area of high concentration to an area of low concentration.

*O*smosis

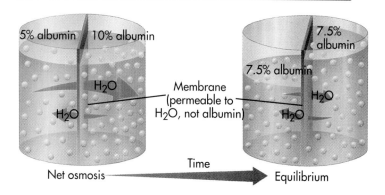

Osmosis is the diffusion of water through a selectively permeable membrane. The membrane shown in the above diagram is permeable to water but not to albumin. Because there are relatively more water molecules in 5% albumin than in 10% albumin, more water molecules osmose from the more dilute into the more concentrated solution (as indicated by the *larger arrow in the left-hand diagram*) than osmose in the opposite direction. The overall direction of osmosis, in other words, is toward the more concentrated solution. Net osmosis produces the following changes in these solutions: their concentrations equilibrate, the volume and the pressure of the originally more concentrated solution increase, and the volume and the pressure of the other solution decrease proportionately.

Effects of Osmosis on Cells

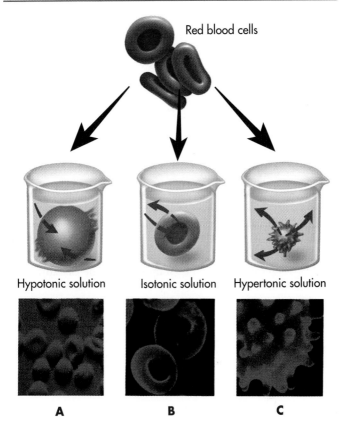

Normal red blood cells **(A)** placed in a hypotonic solution may swell (as the *scanning electron micrograph* shows) or even burst (as the *drawing* shows). Cells placed in an isotonic solution **(B)** maintain a constant volume and pressure because the potential osmotic pressure of the intracellular fluid matches that of the extracellular fluid. Cells placed in a solution that is hypertonic to the intracellular fluid **(C)** lose volume and pressure as water osmoses out of the cell and into the hypertonic solution. The "spikes" seen in the scanning electron micrograph are rigid microtubules of the cytoskeleton. These supports become visible as the cell "deflates."

Determining the Potential Osmotic Pressure of a Solution

Potential osmotic pressure is the maximum osmotic pressure that could develop in a solution if it were separated from distilled water by a selectively permeable membrane. (Actual osmotic pressure is a pressure that already has developed, not just one that could develop.) What determines a solution's potential osmotic pressure? Answer: the number of solute particles in a unit volume of solution directly determines its potential osmotic pressure—the more solute particles per unit volume, the greater the potential osmotic pressure.

If the solute is a nonelectrolyte, the number of solute particles in a liter of solution is determined, as *part A* below indicates, solely by the molar concentration of the solution. (To calculate molar concentration, divide the number of grams of solute in a liter of solution by the molecular weight of the solute.) If the solute is an electrolyte, the number of solute particles per liter is determined by two factors: the molar concentration of the solution and the number of ions formed from each molecule of the electrolyte (see *part B* below).

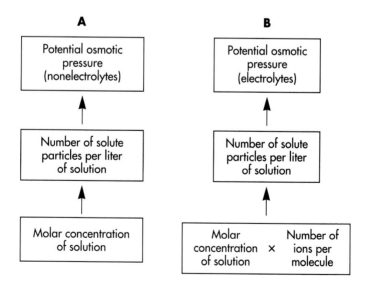

Because the number of solute particles per unit volume directly determines a solution's potential osmotic pressure, one might jump to the conclusion that all solutions having the same percent concentration also have the same potential osmotic pressure. Obviously it is true that all solutions containing the same percent concentration of the same solute do also have the same potential osmotic pressures. All 5% glucose solutions, for example, have a potential osmotic pressure at body temperature of somewhat more than 5,300 mm Hg pressure. But all solutions with the same percent concentrations of different solutes do not have the same molar concentrations. And since it is molar concentration, not percent concentration, that determines potential osmotic pressure, solutions with the same percent concentration of different solutes have different potential osmotic pressures. For example, 5% NaCl at body temperature has a potential osmotic pressure of approximately 33,000 mm Hg—quite different from 5% glucose's potential osmotic pressure of about 5,300 mm Hg. You can calculate these potential osmotic pressures using the formulas given below.

$\mathcal{F}$ormulas for Determining Osmotic Pressure

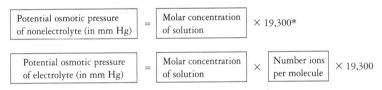

| Potential osmotic pressure of nonelectrolyte (in mm Hg) | = | Molar concentration of solution | × 19,300* |

| Potential osmotic pressure of electrolyte (in mm Hg) | = | Molar concentration of solution | × | Number ions per molecule | × 19,300 |

*Experimentation has shown that a solution with a 1.0 molar concentration of any nonelectrolyte has a potential osmotic pressure of 19,300 mm Hg pressure (at body temperature, 37° C).

| Molar concentration | = | Grams solute in 1 liter solution divided by molecular weight of solute |

Example: Two solutions commonly used in hospitals are 0.85% NaCl and 5% glucose. What is the potential osmotic pressure of 0.85% NaCl at body temperature? (0.85 NaCl = 8.5 gm NaCl in 1 liter solution)
(Molecular weight of NaCl = 58 [NaCl yields two ions per molecule in solution]).

Using the formula given for computing potential osmotic pressure of an electrolyte:

$$\text{Potential osmotic pressure of 0.85\% NaCl} = \frac{8.5}{58} \times 2 \times 19,300 = 5,658.6 \text{ mm Hg pressure}$$

Problem: What is potential osmotic pressure of 5% glucose solution at body temperature? Molecular weight glucose = 180. Glucose does not ionize. It is a nonelectrolyte.†

†5% glucose solution has potential osmotic pressure of 5,359.6 mm Hg pressure.

*C*arrier–Mediated Transport

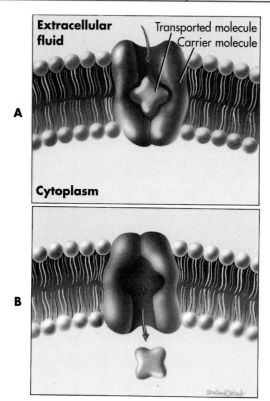

In carrier-mediated transport, a membrane-bound carrier protein attracts a solute molecule to a binding site (illustration **A**) and changes shape in a manner that allows the solute to move to the other side of the membrane (illustration **B**). This type of transport can be passive (driven by a concentration gradient) or active (driven by cellular energy needed to overcome a concentration gradient).

Sodium–Potassium Pump

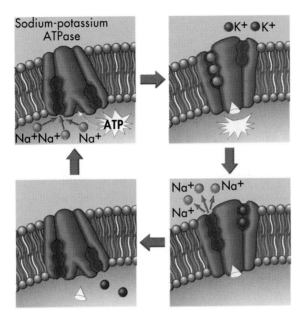

Three sodium (Na^+) ions bind to sodium-binding sites on the carrier's inner face. At the same time, an energy-containing adenosine triphosphate (ATP) molecule produced by the cell's mitochondria binds to the carrier. The ATP breaks apart, transferring its stored energy to the carrier. The carrier then changes shape, releases the three Na^+ ions to the outside of the cell, and attracts two potassium (K^+) ions to its potassium-binding sites. The carrier then returns to its original shape, releasing the two K^+ ions and the remnant of the ATP molecule to the inside of the cell. The carrier is now ready for another pumping cycle.

$\mathscr{E}$ndocytosis

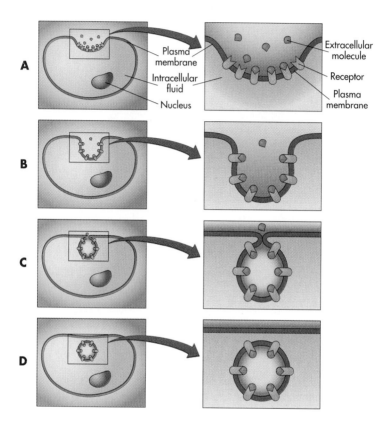

The artist's interpretation shows the basic steps of endocytosis. **A,** Membrane receptors bind to specific molecules in the extracellular fluid. **B,** A portion of the plasma membrane is pulled inward by the cytoskeleton, forming a small pocket around the material to be moved into the cell. **C,** The edges of the pocket eventually fuse, forming a vesicle. **D,** The vesicle is then pulled inward—away from the plasma membrane—by the cytoskeleton. In this example, only the receptor-bound molecules enter the cell. In some cases, some free molecules or even entire cells may also be trapped within the vesicle and transported inward.

*E*nzyme Action

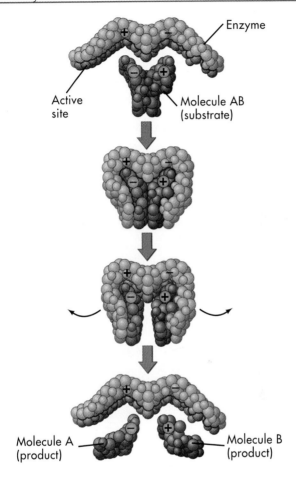

The above illustration is a model of enzyme action. Enzymes are functional proteins whose molecular shape allows them to catalyze chemical reactions. Substrate molecule *AB* is acted on by a digestive enzyme, yielding simpler molecules *A* and *B* as products of the reaction. Notice how the active site of the enzyme chemically fits the substrate—the lock-and-key model of biochemical interaction. Notice also how the enzyme molecule bends its shape in performing its function.

*A*llosteric Effect

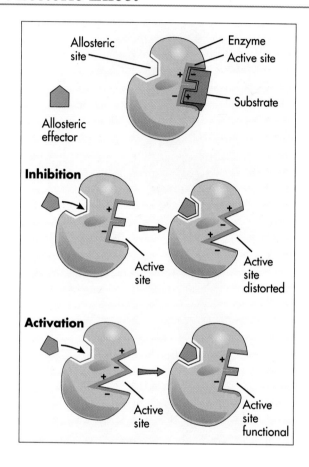

The allosteric effect occurs when some agent, in the case above an allosteric effector molecule, binds to the enzyme at an *allosteric site* and thereby changes the shape of the enzyme's active site. Such an allosteric effect may inhibit enzyme action (by distorting the active site) or activate the enzyme (by giving the active site its functional shape).

Cellular Respiration

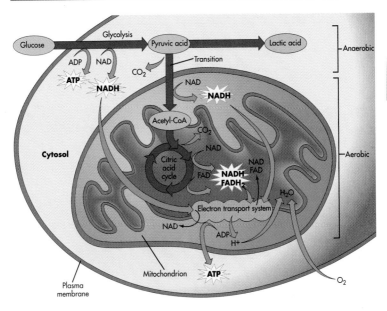

The simplified summary of cellular respiration shown above represents one of the most important catabolic pathways in the cell. Note that one phase (glycolysis) occurs in the cytosol but that the two remaining phases (citric acid cycle and electron transport system) occur within a mitochondrion. Note also the divergence of the anaerobic and aerobic pathways of cellular respiration.

Transcription of Messenger RNA (mRNA)

DNA double helix   mRNA strand

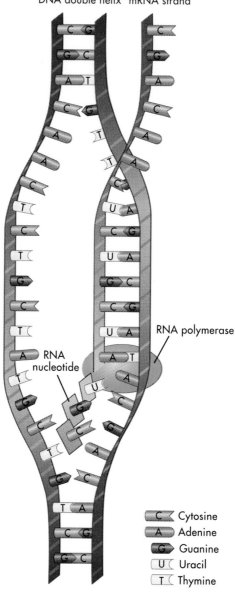

RNA polymerase

RNA nucleotide

C Cytosine
A Adenine
G Guanine
U Uracil
T Thymine

A DNA molecule "unzips" in the region of the gene to be transcribed. RNA nucleotides already present in the nucleus temporarily attach themselves to exposed DNA bases along one strand of the unzipped DNA molecule according to the principle of complementary pairing. As the RNA nucleotides attach to the exposed DNA, they bind to each other, forming a chainlike RNA strand called a *messenger RNA (mRNA)* molecule. Notice in the illustration on p. 64 that the new mRNA strand is an exact copy of the base sequence on the opposite side of the DNA molecule. As in all metabolic processes, the formation of mRNA is controlled by an enzyme—in this case, the enzyme is called *RNA polymerase.*

Protein Synthesis

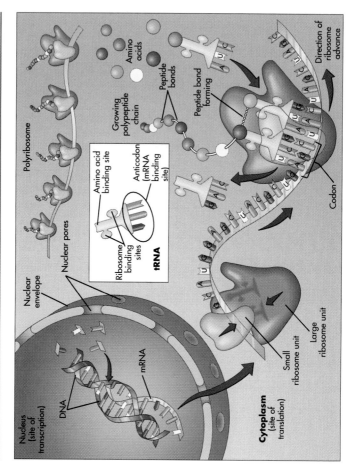

Protein synthesis begins with *transcription*, a process in which an mRNA molecule forms along one gene sequence of a DNA molecule within the cell's nucleus. As it is formed, the mRNA molecule separates from the DNA molecule and leaves the nucleus through the large nuclear pores. Outside the nucleus, ribosome subunits attach to the beginning of the mRNA molecule and begin the process of *translation*. In translation, transfer RNA (tRNA) molecules bring specific amino acids—encoded by each mRNA codon—into place at the ribosome site. As the amino acids are brought into the proper sequence, they are joined together by peptide bonds to form long strands called *polypeptides*. Several polypeptide chains may be needed to make a complete protein molecule.

*S*ummary of Protein Synthesis

Step	Location in the Cell	Description
TRANSCRIPTION		
1	Nucleus	One region, or gene, of a DNA molecule "unzips," exposing its bases.
2	Nucleus	According to the principles of complementary base pairing, RNA nucleotides already present in the nucleoplasm temporarily attach themselves to the exposed bases along one side of the DNA molecule.
3	Nucleus	As RNA nucleotides align themselves along the DNA strand, they bind to each other and thus form a chainlike strand called *messenger RNA (mRNA)*. This binding of RNA nucleotides is controlled by the enzyme RNA polymerase.
PREPARATION OF THE mRNA		
4	Nucleus	As the mRNA strand is formed, it peels away from the DNA strand. The mRNA strand, a copy or *transcript* of a gene, moves out of the nucleus by way of the pores in the nuclear envelope.
5	Cytoplasm	After cellular enzymes "edit" the mRNA molecule by removing portions of the strand, two subunits sandwich the end of the mRNA molecule to form a ribosome.

Step	Location in the Cell	Description
TRANSLATION		
6	Cytoplasm	Specific transfer RNA (tRNA) molecules bring specific amino acids into place at the ribosome, which acts as a sort of "holder" for the mRNA strand and tRNA molecules. The kind of tRNA (and thus, the kind of amino acid) that moves into position is determined by complementary base-pairing: each mRNA codon exposed at the ribosome site will only permit a tRNA with a complementary *anticodon* to attach.
7	Cytoplasm	As each amino acid is brought into place at the ribosome, an enzyme in the ribosome binds it to the amino acid that arrived just before it. The chemical bonds formed, called *peptide bonds,* link the amino acids together to form a long chain called a *polypeptide.*
8	Cytoplasm	As the ribosome moves along the mRNA strand, more and more amino acids are added to the growing polypeptide chain in the sequence dictated by the mRNA codons. (Each codon represents a specific amino acid to be placed in the polypeptide chain.) When the ribosome reaches the end of the mRNA molecule, it drops off the end, separating into large and small subunits again. Often, enzymes later link two or more polypeptides together to form a whole protein molecule.

*L*ife Cycle of the Cell

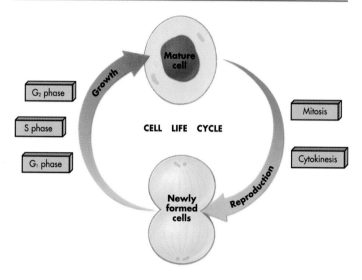

The processes of growth and reproduction of successive generations of cells exhibit a cyclic pattern. Newly formed cells grow to maturity by synthesizing new molecules and organelles (G_1 and G_2 phases), including the replication of an extra set of DNA molecules in anticipation of reproduction (*S phase*). Mature cells reproduce by first distributing the two identical sets of DNA (produced during the growth phase) in the orderly process of *mitosis*, then by splitting the plasma membrane, cytoplasm, and organelles of the parent cell into two distinct daughter cells (*cytokinesis*).

*D*NA Replication

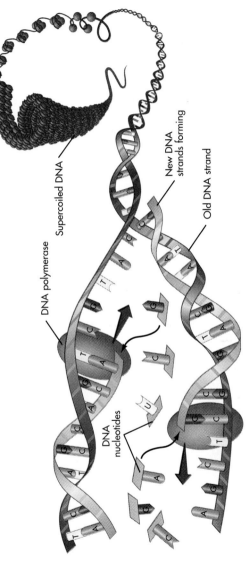

DNA polymerase

Supercoiled DNA

New DNA strands forming

Old DNA strand

DNA nucleotides

When a DNA molecule makes a copy of itself, it "unzips" to expose its nucleotide bases. Through the mechanism of obligatory base-pairing, coordinated by the enzyme *DNA polymerase*, new DNA nucleotides bind to the exposed bases. This forms a new "other half" to each half of the original molecule. After all the bases have new nucleotides bound to them, two identical DNA molecules will be ready for distribution to the two daughter cells.

*S*ummary of DNA Replication

Step	Description
1	DNA molecules uncoil and "unzip," exposing their bases.
2	Nucleotides already present in the intracellular fluid of the nucleus attach to the exposed bases according to the principle of obligatory base-pairing.
3	As nucleotides attach to complementary bases along each DNA strand, the enzyme *DNA polymerase* causes them to bind to each other.
4	As new nucleotides fill in the spaces left open on each DNA strand, two identical *daughter molecules* are formed. As the parent DNA molecule completely unzips, the two daughter molecules coil to become distinct, but genetically identical, DNA double helices called *chromatids*.

The Major Events of Mitosis

Prophase	Metaphase	Anaphase	Telophase
1. Chromosomes shorten and thicken (from coiling of DNA molecules that compose them); each chromosome consists of two chromatids attached at centromere 2. Centrioles move to opposite poles of cell; spindle fibers appear and begin to orient between opposing poles 3. Nucleoli and nuclear membrane disappear	1. Chromosomes align across equator of spindle fibers; each pair of chromatids attached to spindle fiber at its centromere	1. Each centromere splits, thereby detaching two chromatids that compose each chromosome each from each other 2. Sister chromatids (now called chromosomes) move to opposite poles; there are now twice as many chromosomes as there were before mitosis started	1. Changes occurring during telophase essentially reverse of those taking place during prophase; new chromosomes start elongating (DNA molecules start uncoiling) 2. Nuclear envelope reappears, enclosing each new set of chromosomes 3. Spindle fibers disappear

Centrioles

Nucleus

Chromatids

Centromere

Spindle fibers

Sister chromatids

Nuclear envelope

*S*ummary of Cell Life Cycle

Phase of Cell Life Cycle	Description	Phase of Cell Life Cycle	Description
CELL GROWTH			
Protein synthesis	Proteins are manufactured according to the cell's genetic code; functional proteins, the enzymes, direct the synthesis of other molecules in the cells and thus the production of more and larger organelles and plasma membrane; sometimes called the *first growth phase* or G_1 *phase* of interphase	Protein synthesis	After DNA is replicated, the cell continues to grow by means of protein synthesis and the resulting synthesis of other molecules and various organelles; this *second growth phase* is also called the G_2 *phase*
		CELL REPRODUCTION	
DNA replication	Nucleotides, influenced by newly synthe-sized enzymes, arrange themselves along the open sides of an "unzipped" DNA molecule, thereby creating two identical daughter DNA molecules; produces two identical sets of the cell's genetic code, enabling the cell to later split into two different cells, each with its own com-plete set of DNA; sometimes called the {DNA} *synthesis stage* or *S phase* of interphase	Mitosis or meiosis	The parent cell's replicated set of DNA is divided into two sets and separated by an orderly process into distinct cell nuclei; mitosis subdivided into at least four phases: *prophase, metaphase, anaphase,* and *telophase*
		Cytokinesis	The plasma membrane of the parent cell "pinches in," eventually separating the cytoplasm and two daughter nuclei into two genetically identical daughter cells

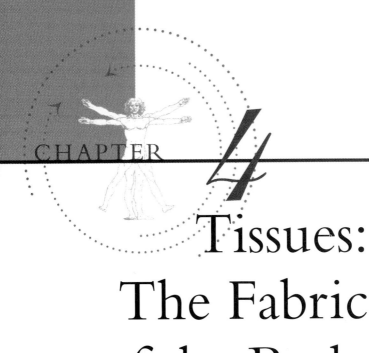

CHAPTER 4

Tissues: The Fabric of the Body

A tissue is a group of similar cells that perform a common function. Each tissue specializes in performing at least one unique function that helps maintain homeostasis, assuring the survival of the whole body. Regardless of the size, shape, or arrangement of cells in a tissue, they are all surrounded by or embedded in a nonliving intercellular material that is often simply called *matrix*.

All tissues in the human body can be classified by their structure and function into four principal types: (1) epithelial, (2) connective, (3) muscle tissue, and (4) nervous tissue. These tissue types originate from the three primary germ layers.

Primary Germ Layers

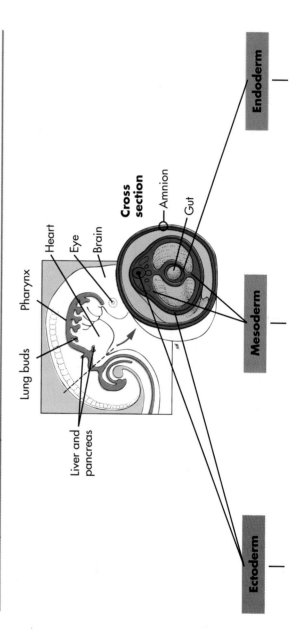

Pharynx

Heart

Eye

Brain

Lung buds

Liver and
pancreas

**Cross
section**

Amnion

Gut

Endoderm

Mesoderm

Ectoderm

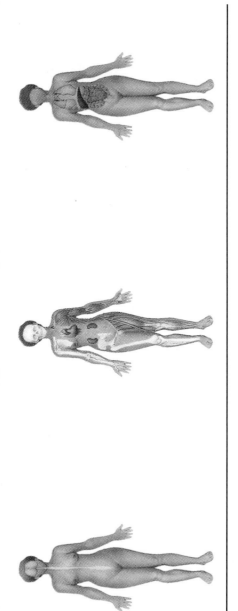

ECTODERM

Epithelium (epidermis) of skin
Lining of mouth, anus, nostrils
Sweat and sebaceous glands
Epidermal derivatives (hair, enamel of teeth)
Nervous system (brain and spinal cord)
Epithelial (sensory) parts of eyes, nose, ear

MESODERM

Muscles
Skeleton (bones and cartilage)
Blood
Epithelial lining of blood vessels
Dermis of skin and dentin of teeth
Organs (except lining) of excretory and reproductive systems
Connective tissue

ENDODERM

Epithelium (lining) of digestive and respiratory systems
Secretory parts of liver and pancreas
Urinary bladder
Epithelial lining of urethra
Thyroid, parathyroid, thymus

The illustration above shows the primary germ layers and the body systems into which they develop. The structures derived from the primary germ layers are listed below each figure.

Classification of Epithelial Tissues

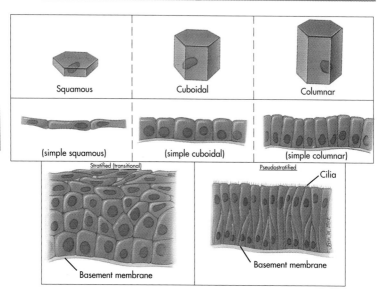

Squamous	Cuboidal	Columnar
(simple squamous)	(simple cuboidal)	(simple columnar)

Stratified (transitional)

Pseudostratified

Cilia

Basement membrane

Basement membrane

Epithelial tissues are classified according to the shape and arrangement of cells. The color scheme of the above drawings is based on a common staining technique used by histologists called *hematoxylin and eosin (H&E) staining*. H&E staining usually renders the cytoplasm pink and the chromatin inside the nucleus a purplish color. The cellular membranes, including the plasma membrane and nuclear envelope, usually do not pick up any stain and thus are transparent.

$\mathscr{S}$imple Squamous Epithelium

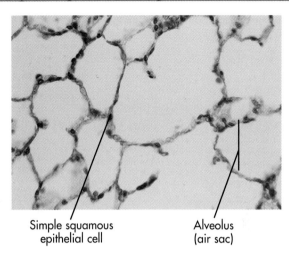

Simple squamous
epithelial cell

Alveolus
(air sac)

A photomicrograph of lung tissue shows thin simple squamous epithelium lining the tiny air sacs of the lung. Notice how the H&E staining renders the cytoplasm of each cell pink and each nucleus a purplish color.

$\mathscr{C}$lassification Scheme for Membranous Epithelial Tissues

	Shape of Cells*	Tissue Type
One layer	Squamous	Simple squamous
	Cuboidal	Simple cuboidal
	Columnar	Simple columnar
	Pseudostratified columnar	Pseudostratified columnar
Several layers	Squamous	Stratified squamous
	Cuboidal	Stratified cuboidal
	Columnar	Stratified columnar
	(Varies)	Transitional

*In the top layer (if more than one layer in the tissue).

Simple Cuboidal Epithelium

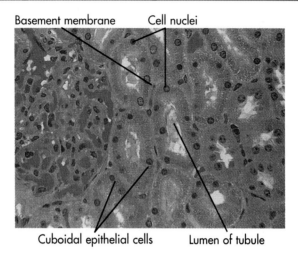

Basement membrane   Cell nuclei

Cuboidal epithelial cells   Lumen of tubule

A photomicrograph of kidney tubules shows the single layer of cuboidal cells touching a basement membrane.

Simple Columnar Epithelium

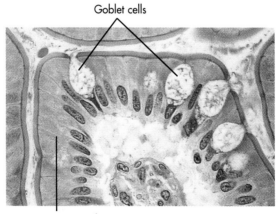

Goblet cells

Columnar epithelial cell

A photomicrograph of simple columnar epithelium is shown above. Note the goblet, or mucus-producing, cells present.

*P*seudostratified Ciliated Epithelium

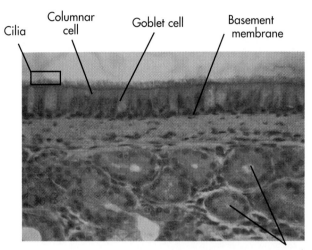

Cilia   Columnar cell   Goblet cell   Basement membrane

Mucous glands

The above photomicrograph of the trachea shows that each irregularly shaped columnar cell touches the underlying basement membrane. Placement of cell nuclei at irregular levels in the cells gives a false (pseudo) impression of stratification.

*S*tratified Squamous (Keratinized) Epithelium

Cornified layer

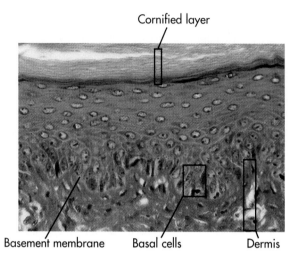

Basement membrane   Basal cells   Dermis

A photomicrograph of the skin shows cells becoming progressively flattened and scalelike as they approach the surface and are lost. The cornified layer is made up of completely keratinized cells.

Stratified Squamous (Nonkeratinized) Epithelium

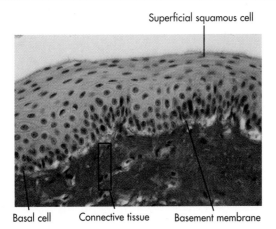

Superficial squamous cell

Basal cell   Connective tissue   Basement membrane

In the above photomicrograph of vaginal tissue, each cell in the layer is flattened near the surface and attached to the sheet. No flaking of dead (keratinized) cells from the surface occurs. All cells have nuclei.

Transitional Epithelium

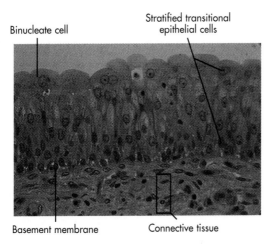

Binucleate cell   Stratified transitional epithelial cells

Basement membrane   Connective tissue

The above photomicrograph of the urinary bladder shows that cell shape is variable from cuboidal to squamous. Several layers of cells are present. Intermediate and surface cells do not touch the basement membrane.

Structural Classification of Multicellular Exocrine Glands

Shape*	Complexity†		Type	Example
Tubular (single, straight)	Simple	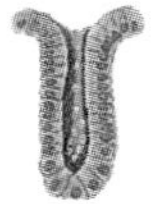	Simple tubular	Intestinal glands
Tubular (coiled)	Simple	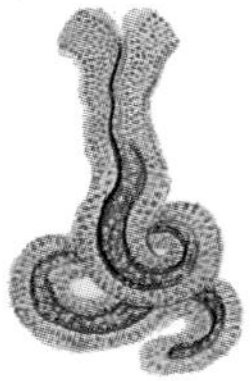	Simple coiled tubular	Sweat glands
Tubular (multiple)	Simple	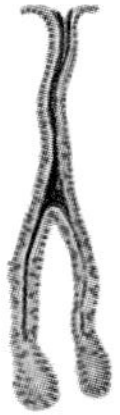	Simple branched tubular	Gastric (stomach) glands
Alveolar (single)	Simple	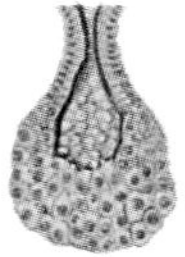	Simple alveolar	Sebaceous (skin oil) glands

†	*		Gland type	Example
Simple	Alveolar (multiple)		Simple branched alveolar	Sebaceous glands
Compound	Tubular (multiple)		Compound tubular	Mammary glands
Compound	Alveolar (multiple)		Compound alveolar	Mammary glands
Compound	Some tubular; some alveolar		Compound tubuloalveolar	Salivary glands

*Shape of the distal, secreting units of the gland.
†Number of ducts *reaching the surface.*

*T*he Location and Function of Tissues

Tissue	Location	Function
EPITHELIAL		
Membranous		
Simple squamous	Alveoli of lungs	Absorption by diffusion of respiratory gases between alveolar air and blood
	Lining of blood and lymphatic vessels (called endothelium: classified as connective tissue by some histologists)	Absorption by diffusion, filtration, osmosis
	Surface layer of pleura, pericardium, peritoneum (called mesothelium; classified as connective tissue by some histologists)	Absorption by diffusion and osmosis; also, secretion
Stratified squamous	Surface of mucous membrane lining mouth, esophagus, and vagina	Protection
	Surface of skin (epidermis)	Protection
Transitional	Surface of mucous membrane lining urinary bladder and ureters	Permits stretching
Simple columnar	Surface layer of mucous lining of stomach, intestines, and part of respiratory tract	Protection; secretion; absorption; moving of mucus (by ciliated columnar epithelium)
Stratified columnar	Lining of portions of the male urethra; mucous membrane near anus (rare)	Protection
Pseudostratified columnar	Surface of mucous membrane lining trachea, large bronchi, nasal mucosa, and parts of male reproductive tract (epididymis and vas deferens); lines large ducts of some glands (e.g., parotid)	Protection

Tissue	Location	Function
Simple cuboidal	Ducts and tubules of many organs, including exocrine glands and kidneys	Secretion; absorption
Stratified cuboidal	Ducts of sweat glands; lining of pharynx; covering portion of epiglottis	Protection
Glandular	Glands	Secretion
CONNECTIVE		
Fibrous		
Loose, ordinary (areolar)	Between other tissues and organs	Connection
	Superficial fascia	Connection
	Under skin	Protection
Adipose (fat)	Padding at various points	Insulation
		Support
		Reserve food
Reticular	Inner framework of spleen, lymph nodes, bone marrow	Support
		Filtration
Dense fibrous		
Regular	Tendons	Flexible but strong connection
	Ligaments	
	Aponeuroses	
Irregular	Deep fascia	Connection
	Dermis	Support
	Scars	
	Capsule of kidney, etc.	

Continued

The Location and Function of Tissues—cont'd

Tissue	Location	Function
Bone	Skeleton	Support
		Protection
		Calcium reservoir
Cartilage		
Hyaline	Part of nasal septum	Firm but flexible support
	Covering articular surfaces of bones	
	Larynx	
	Rings in trachea and bronchi	
Fibrocartilage	Disks between vertebrae	
	Symphysis pubis	
Elastic	External ear	
	Eustachian tube	
Blood	In the blood vessels	Transportation
		Protection

MUSCLE		
Skeletal (striated voluntary)	Muscles that attach to bones	Movement of bones
	Extrinsic eyeball muscles	Eye movements
	Upper third of esophagus	First part of swallowing
Smooth (nonstriated, involuntary, or visceral)	In walls of tubular viscera of digestive, respiratory, and genitourinary tracts	Movement of substances along respective tracts
	In walls of blood vessels and large lymphatic vessels	Change diameter of blood vessels, thereby aiding in regulation of blood pressure
	In ducts of glands	Movement of substances along ducts
	Intrinsic eye muscles (iris and ciliary body)	Change diameter of pupils and shape of lens
	Arrector muscles of hairs	Erection of hairs (gooseflesh)
Cardiac (striated involuntary)	Wall of heart	Contraction of heart
NERVOUS		
	Brain	Excitability
	Spinal cord	Conduction
	Nerves	

Loose, Ordinary (Areolar) Connective Tissue

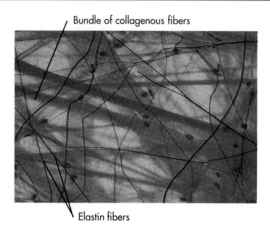

Bundle of collagenous fibers

Elastin fibers

In the photomicrograph above, notice how the H&E staining renders the bundles of collagen fibers a pinkish color and the elastin fibers and cell nuclei a purplish color. The arrangement of the fibers is loose compared to fibers in dense fibrous connective tissue.

Adipose Tissue

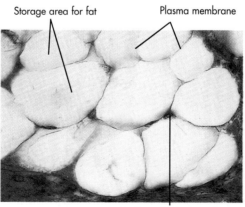

Storage area for fat   Plasma membrane

Nucleus of adipose cell

Adipose tissue cells have large storage spaces for fat inside of them.

$\mathscr{R}$eticular Connective Tissue

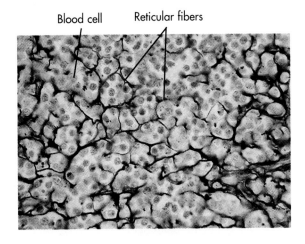

The supporting framework of reticular fibers is *stained black* in the above photomicrograph of a section of spleen tissue.

$\mathscr{D}$ense Fibrous (Regular) Connective Tissue

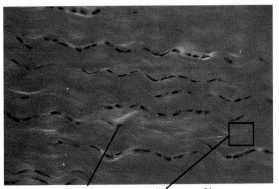

The photomicrograph of tissue in a tendon shows multiple bundles of collagenous fibers arranged in parallel (regular) rows.

$\mathscr{D}$ense Fibrous (Irregular) Connective Tissue

Fibroblast   Collagenous fibers

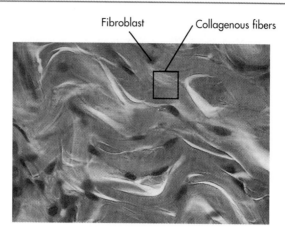

The above photomicrograph of a section of skin (dermis) shows irregular arrangements of collagenous fibers (*pink*) and purple-staining fibroblast cell nuclei.

$\mathscr{B}$one Tissue

Osteon (Haversian system)

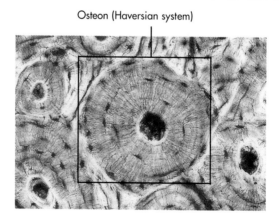

The photomicrograph of dried, ground bone shows many wheel-like structural units of bone, known as *osteons* or *Haversian systems.*

Hyaline Cartilage

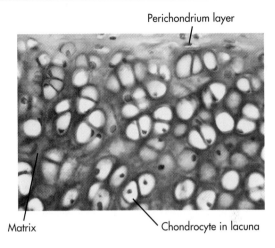

Perichondrium layer

Matrix

Chondrocyte in lacuna

The photomicrograph of the trachea shows many spaces, or lacunae, in the gel-like matrix.

Fibrocartilage

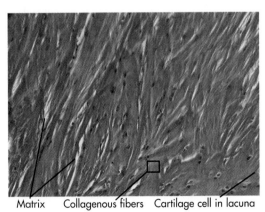

Matrix   Collagenous fibers   Cartilage cell in lacuna

The photomicrograph above of the pubic symphysis joint shows dense fibers that fill the matrix and convey shock–absorbing qualities.

Elastic Cartilage

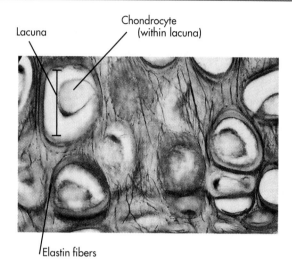

Lacuna

Chondrocyte (within lacuna)

Elastin fibers

In the above photomicrograph, the cartilage cells in the lacunae are surrounded by matrix and dark-staining elastin fibers.

Blood

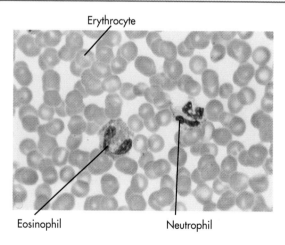

Erythrocyte

Eosinophil

Neutrophil

The photomicrograph of a human blood smear shows two white blood cells, or leukocytes, surrounded by numerous smaller red blood cells.

Skeletal Muscle

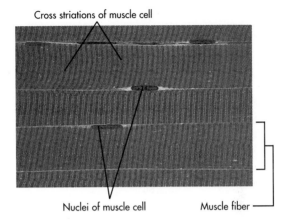

Cross striations of muscle cell

Nuclei of muscle cell   Muscle fiber

The photomicrograph above shows striations of the muscle cell fibers in longitudinal section.

Smooth Muscle

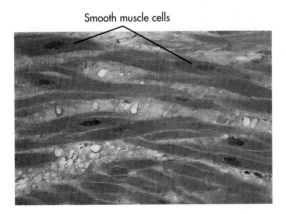

Smooth muscle cells

The photomicrograph of a longitudinal section of smooth muscle shows central placement of the nuclei in the spindle-shaped smooth muscle fibers.

Cardiac Muscle

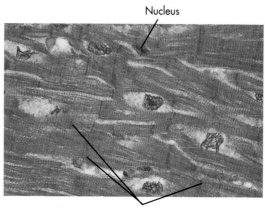

Nucleus

Intercalated disks

In the photomicrograph above, the dark bands, called *intercalated disks,* which are characteristic of cardiac muscle, are easily identified in this tissue section.

Nervous Tissue

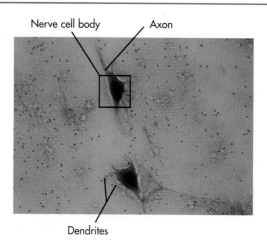

Nerve cell body   Axon

Dendrites

The micrograph shows multipolar neurons in a smear of spinal cord. Both neurons in this slide show characteristic soma, or cell bodies, and multiple cell processes.

Types of Body Membranes

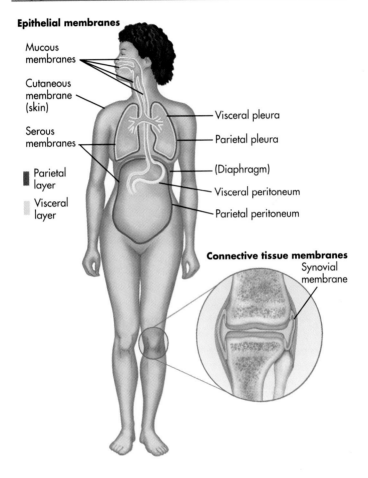

Epithelial membranes

Mucous membranes

Cutaneous membrane (skin)

Serous membranes

■ Parietal layer

▫ Visceral layer

Visceral pleura

Parietal pleura

(Diaphragm)

Visceral peritoneum

Parietal peritoneum

Connective tissue membranes
Synovial membrane

The cutaneous membrane, or skin, covers body surfaces that are exposed to the external environment. It is the primary organ of the integumentary system and one of the most important and certainly one of the largest and most visible organs of the body.

Serous membrane lines cavities that are not open to the external environment and covers many of the organs inside these cavities. Like all epithelial membranes, a serous membrane is composed of two distinct layers of tissue. The *parietal membrane* is the portion that lines the wall of the cavity like wallpaper; the *visceral membrane* covers the surface of the viscera (organs within the cavity).

Mucous membranes are epithelial membranes that line body surfaces opening directly to the exterior. Examples include those lining the respiratory, digestive, urinary, and reproductive tracts. Mucous membranes get their name from the fact that they produce a film of mucus that coats and protects the underlying cells.

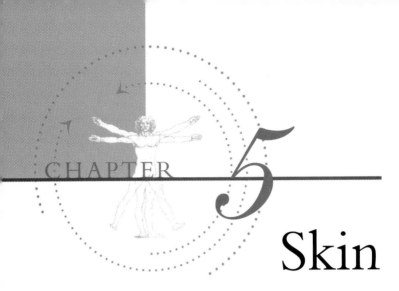

CHAPTER 5

Skin

The skin forms a self-repairing and protective boundary between the internal environment of the body and an often hostile external world. Integument is another name for the skin; integumentary system is a term used to denote the skin and its appendages—hair, nails, and skin glands.

The skin is a thin, relatively flat organ classified as a membrane—the cutaneous membrane. Two main layers compose the skin: an outer, thinner layer called the *epidermis* and an inner, thicker layer named the *dermis*.

*M*icroscopic Diagram of the Skin

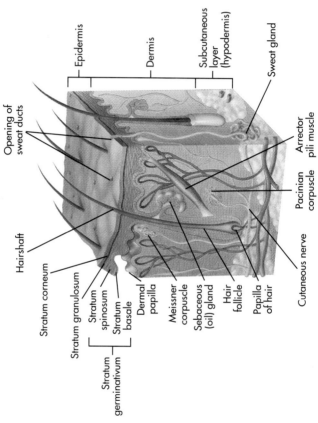

The epidermis, shown in longitudinal section, is raised at one corner to reveal the ridges in the dermis.

Functions of the Skin

Function	Example	Mechanism
Protection	From micro-organisms	Surface film/mechanical barrier
	From dehydration	Keratin
	From ultraviolet radiation	Melanin
	From mechanical trauma	Tissue strength
Sensation	Pain	Somatic sensory receptors
	Heat and cold	
	Pressure	
	Touch	
Permits movement and growth without injury	Body growth and change in body contours during movement	Elastic and recoil properties of skin and subcutaneous tissue
Endocrine	Vitamin D production	Activation of precursor compound in skin cells by ultraviolet light
Excretion	Water	Regulation of sweat volume and content
	Urea	
	Ammonia	
	Uric acid	
Immunity	Destruction of microorganisms and interaction with immune system cells (helper T cells)	Phagocytic cells and Langerhans cells
Temperature regulation	Heat loss or retention	Regulation of blood flow to the skin and evaporation of sweat

*G*rowth and Repair of the Skin

LANGER'S (CLEAVAGE) LINES. The dense bundles of white collagenous fibers that characterize the reticular layer of the dermis tend to orient themselves in patterns that differ in appearance from one body area to another. The result is formation of patterns called *Langer's lines,* or *cleavage lines.*

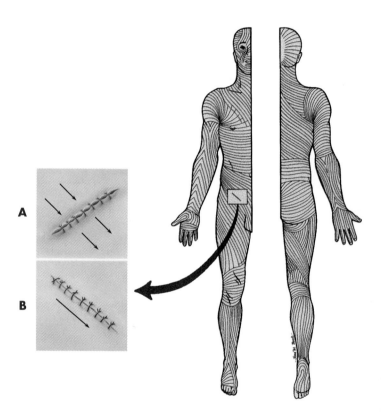

If an incision "cuts across" cleavage lines (**A**), stress tends to pull the cut edges apart and may retard healing. Surgical incisions that are parallel to cleavage lines (**B**) are subjected to less stress and tend to heal more rapidly.

RULE OF NINES. When the skin is burned, treatment and prognosis for recovery depend in large part on total area involved and severity of the burn.

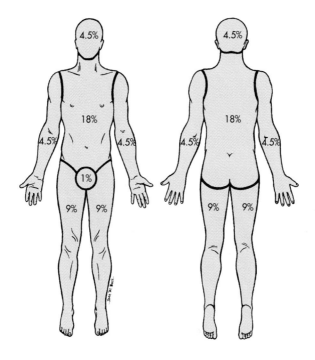

"Rule of nines" is one method used to estimate amount of skin surface burned in an adult.

*A*ppendages of the Skin

HAIR FOLLICLE

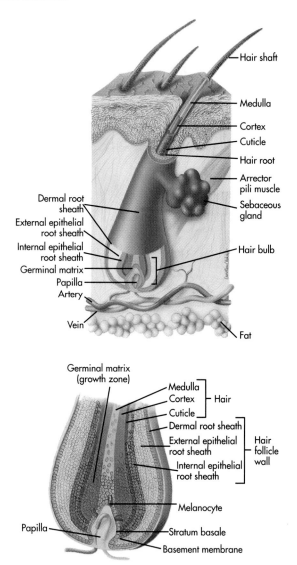

This illustration shows the relationship of a hair follicle and related structures to the epidermal and dermal layers of the skin. The enlargement on the right shows a hair follicle wall and hair bulb.

Structure of Nails

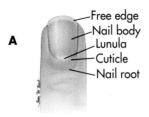

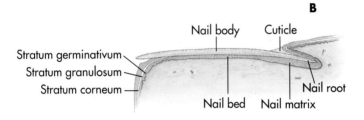

This illustration shows a fingernail as viewed from above (**A**) and also a sagittal section of the fingernail and associated structures (**B**).

6

Skeletal System

Structurally there are four types of bones in the human skeleton: long bones, short bones, flat bones, and irregular bones. Bones differ in size and shape and also in the amount and proportion of two different types of bone tissue that comprise them: *compact bone*, solid in appearance, and *cancellous*, or spongy, *bone*.

𝒫arts of a Long Bone

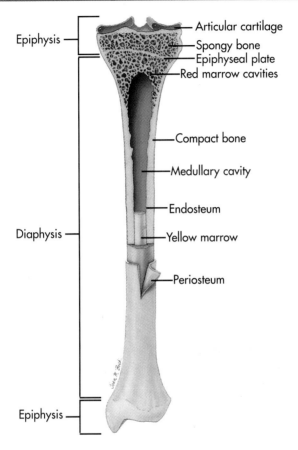

Epiphysis

Articular cartilage
Spongy bone
Epiphyseal plate
Red marrow cavities

Compact bone

Medullary cavity

Endosteum

Diaphysis

Yellow marrow

Periosteum

Epiphysis

Longitudinal section of the tibia.

𝒮tructure of Compact and Cancellous Bone

Compact bone contains many cylinder-shaped structural units called *osteons*, or *Haversian systems*. Cancellous bone has no osteons; instead, it consists of needlelike bony spicules called *trabeculae*.

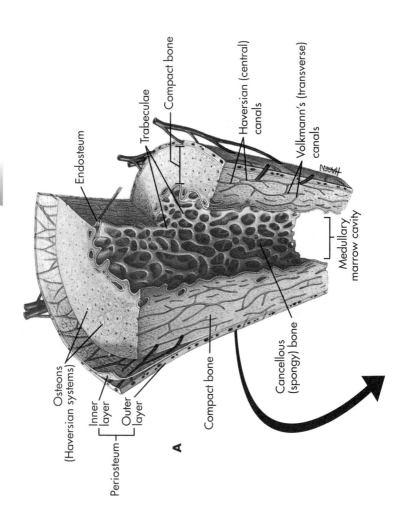

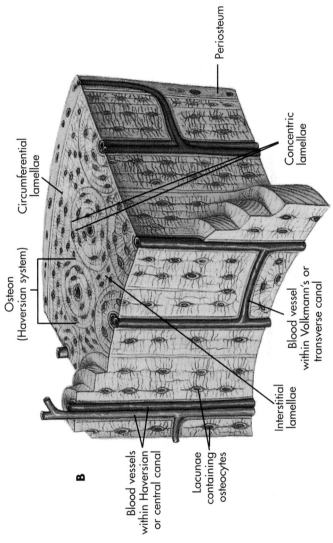

Periosteum

Concentric
lamellae

Circumferential
lamellae

Osteon
(Haversian system)

Blood vessel
within Volkmann's or
transverse canal

Interstitial
lamellae

B

Blood vessels
within Haversian
or central canal

Lacunae
containing
osteocytes

The longitudinal section of long bone (**A**) shows both cancellous and compact bone. The magnified section (**B**) is a view of compact bone.

ℋuman Skeleton

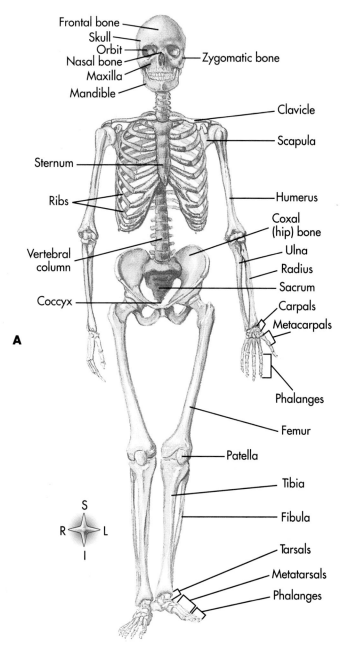

Frontal bone
Skull
Orbit
Nasal bone
Maxilla
Mandible
Zygomatic bone
Clavicle
Scapula
Sternum
Ribs
Humerus
Coxal (hip) bone
Vertebral column
Ulna
Radius
Sacrum
Coccyx
Carpals
Metacarpals
Phalanges
Femur
Patella
Tibia
Fibula
Tarsals
Metatarsals
Phalanges

S
R — L
I

A

Anterior **(A)** and posterior **(B)** views of the human skeleton.

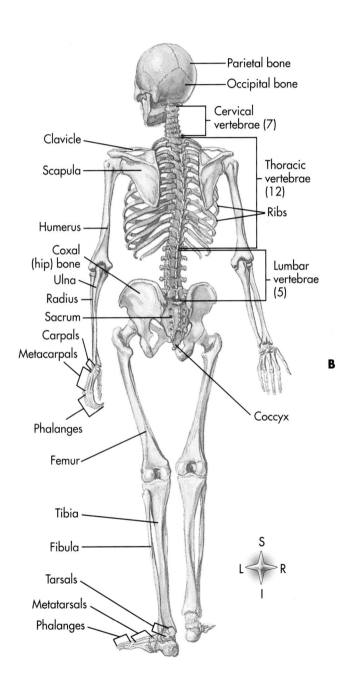

Parietal bone
Occipital bone
Cervical vertebrae (7)
Clavicle
Scapula
Thoracic vertebrae (12)
Ribs
Humerus
Coxal (hip) bone
Ulna
Radius
Lumbar vertebrae (5)
Sacrum
Carpals
Metacarpals
Phalanges
Coccyx
Femur
Tibia
Fibula
Tarsals
Metatarsals
Phalanges

B

S
L R
I

$\mathscr{B}$ones of the Skeleton (206 Total)*

Part of Body	Name of Bone
AXIAL SKELETON (80 BONES TOTAL)	
Skull (28 bones total)	
Cranium (8 bones)	Frontal (1)
	Parietal (2)
	Temporal (2)
	Occipital (1)
	Sphenoid (1)
	Ethmoid (1)
Face (14 bones)	Nasal (2)
	Maxillary (2)
	Zygomatic (malar) (2)
	Mandible (1)
	Lacrimal (2)
	Palatine (2)
	Inferior conchae (turbinates) (2)
	Vomer (1)
Ear bones (6 bones)	Malleus (hammer) (2)
	Incus (anvil) (2)
	Stapes (stirrup) (2)
Hyoid bone (1)	
Spinal Column	
(26 bones total)	Cervical vertebrae (7)
	Thoracic vertebrae (12)
	Lumbar vertebrae (5)
	Sacrum (1)
	Coccyx (1)
Sternum and ribs	Sternum (1)
(25 bones total)	True ribs (14)
	False ribs (10)

*An inconstant number of small, flat, round bones known as sesamoid bones (because of their resemblance to sesame seeds) are found in various tendons in which considerable pressure develops. Because the number of these bones varies greatly between individuals, only two of them, the patellae, have been counted among the 206 bones of the body. Generally, two of them can be found in each thumb (in flexor tendon near metacarpophalangeal and interphalangeal joints) and great toe plus several others in the upper and lower extremities. Wormian bones, the small islets of bone frequently found in some of the cranial sutures, have not been counted in this list of 206 bones because of their variable occurrence.

Part of Body	Name of Bone
APPENDICULAR SKELETON (126 BONES TOTAL)	
Upper extremities	
(including shoulder girdle)	Clavicle (2)
(64 bones total)	Scapula (2)
	Humerus (2)
	Radius (2)
	Ulna (2)
	Carpals (16)
	Metacarpals (10)
	Phalanges (28)
Lower extremities	
(including hip girdle)	Coxal bones (2)
(62 bones total)	Femur (2)
	Patella (2)
	Tibia (2)
	Fibula (2)
	Tarsals (14)
	Metatarsals (10)
	Phalanges (28)

*T*erms Used to Describe Bone Markings

Term	Meaning
Angle	A corner
Body	The main portion of a bone
Condyle	Rounded bump; usually fits into a fossa on another bone, forming a joint
Crest	Moderately raised ridge; generally a site for muscle attachment
Epicondyle	Bump near a condyle; often gives the appearance of a "bump on a bump"; for muscle attachment
Facet	Flat surface that forms a joint with another facet or flat bone
Fissure	Long, cracklike hole for blood vessels and nerves
Foramen	Round hole for vessels and nerves (pl. foramina)
Fossa	Depression; often receives an articulating bone (pl. fossae)
Head	Distinct epiphysis on a long bone, separated from the shaft by a narrowed portion (or neck)
Line	Similar to a crest but not raised as much (is often rather faint)
Margin	Edge of a flat bone or flat portion of edge of a flat area
Meatus	Tubelike opening or channel (pl. meati)
Neck	A narrowed portion, usually at the base of a head
Notch	A V-like depression in the margin or edge of a flat area
Process	A raised area or projection
Ramus	Curved portion of a bone, like a ram's horn (pl. rami)
Sinus	Cavity within a bone
Spine	Similar to a crest but raised more; a sharp, pointed process; for muscle attachment
Sulcus	Groove or elongated depression (pl. sulci)
Trochanter	Large bump for muscle attachment (larger than tubercle or tuberosity)
Tuberosity	Oblong, raised bump, usually for muscle attachment, small tuberosity is called a *tubercle*

$\mathscr{A}$nterior View of the Skull

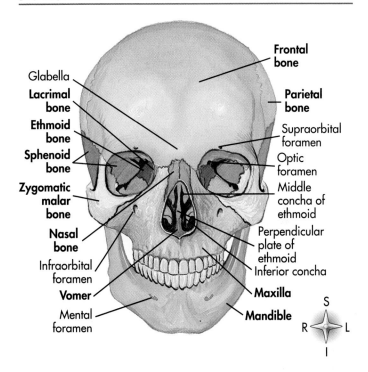

Glabella

Lacrimal bone

Ethmoid bone

Sphenoid bone

Zygomatic malar bone

Nasal bone

Infraorbital foramen

Vomer

Mental foramen

Frontal bone

Parietal bone

Supraorbital foramen

Optic foramen

Middle concha of ethmoid

Perpendicular plate of ethmoid

Inferior concha

Maxilla

Mandible

S

R — L

I

Skull Viewed From the Right Side

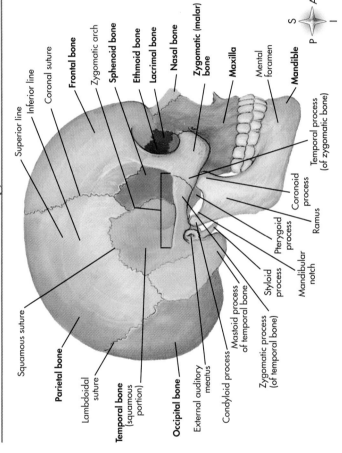

Squamous suture

Superior line

Inferior line

Coronal suture

Frontal bone

Zygomatic arch

Sphenoid bone

Ethmoid bone

Lacrimal bone

Nasal bone

Zygomatic (malar) bone

Maxilla

Mental foramen

Mandible

Temporal process (of zygomatic bone)

Coronoid process

Ramus

Pterygoid process

Mandibular notch

Styloid process

Zygomatic process (of temporal bone)

Mastoid process of temporal bone

Condyloid process

External auditory meatus

Occipital bone

Temporal bone (squamous portion)

Lambdoidal suture

Parietal bone

S

P

A

I

Floor of the Cranial Cavity

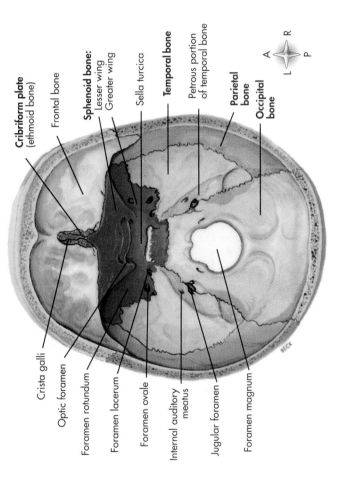

Cribriform plate
(ethmoid bone)

Frontal bone

Sphenoid bone:
Lesser wing
Greater wing

Sella turcica

Temporal bone

Petrous portion
of temporal bone

**Parietal
bone**

**Occipital
bone**

Crista galli

Optic foramen

Foramen rotundum

Foramen lacerum

Foramen ovale

Internal auditory
meatus

Jugular foramen

Foramen magnum

A
R
L
P

BECK

Skull Viewed From Below

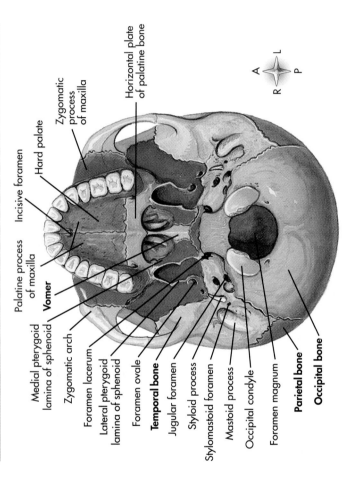

Palatine process of maxilla

Incisive foramen

Hard palate

Zygomatic process of maxilla

Horizontal plate of palatine bone

Palatine process of maxilla

Vomer

Medial pterygoid lamina of sphenoid

Zygomatic arch

Foramen lacerum

Lateral pterygoid lamina of sphenoid

Foramen ovale

Temporal bone

Jugular foramen

Styloid process

Stylomastoid foramen

Mastoid process

Occipital condyle

Foramen magnum

Parietal bone

Occipital bone

A
R — L
P

Left Half of the Skull Viewed From Within

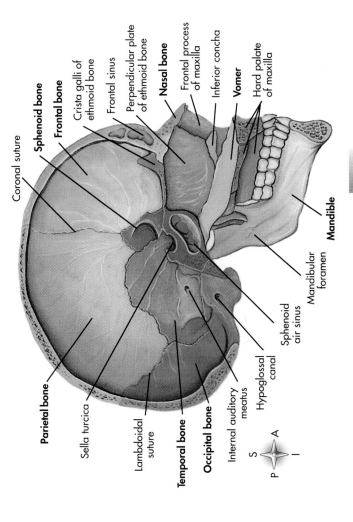

Coronal suture

Sphenoid bone

Frontal bone

Crista galli of ethmoid bone

Frontal sinus

Perpendicular plate of ethmoid bone

Nasal bone

Frontal process of maxilla

Inferior concha

Vomer

Hard palate of maxilla

Mandible

Parietal bone

Sella turcica

Lambdoidal suture

Temporal bone

Occipital bone

Internal auditory meatus

Hypoglossal canal

Sphenoid air sinus

Mandibular foramen

S
P — A
I

$\mathcal{B}$ones That Form the Left Orbit of the Skull

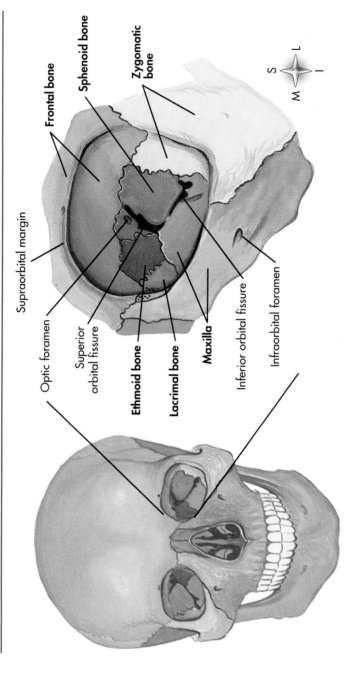

Frontal bone

Sphenoid bone

Zygomatic bone

Supraorbital margin

Optic foramen

Superior orbital fissure

Ethmoid bone

Lacrimal bone

Maxilla

Inferior orbital fissure

Infraorbital foramen

S
M — L
I

Cranial Bones and Their Markings

Bones and Markings	Description
FRONTAL	Forehead bone; also forms most of roof of orbits (eye sockets) and anterior part of cranial floor
Supraorbital margin	Arched ridge just below eyebrow, forms upper edge of orbit
Frontal sinuses	Cavities inside bone just above supraorbital margin; lined with mucosa; contain air
Frontal tuberosities	Bulge above each orbit; most prominent part of forehead
Superciliary ridges	Ridges caused by projection of frontal sinuses; eyebrows lie superficial to these ridges
Supraorbital foramen (sometimes notch)	Foramen or notch in supraorbital margin slightly medial to its midpoint; transmits supraorbital nerve and blood vessels
Glabella	Smooth area between superciliary ridges and above nose
PARIETAL	Prominent, bulging bones behind frontal bone; forms top sides of cranial cavity
SPHENOID	Keystone of cranial floor; forms its midportion; resembles bat with wings outstretched and legs extended downward posteriorly; lies behind and slightly above nose and throat; forms part of floor and sidewalls of orbit
Body	Hollow, cubelike central portion
Greater wings	Lateral projections from body, form part of outer wall of orbit
Lesser wings	Thin, triangular projections from upper part of sphenoid body; form posterior part of roof of orbit
Sella turcica (or *Turk's saddle*)	Saddle-shaped depression on upper surface of sphenoid body; contains pituitary gland
Sphenoid sinuses	Irregular mucosa-lined, air-filled spaces within central part of sphenoid
Pterygoid processes	Downward projections on either side where body and greater wing unite; comparable to extended legs of bat if entire bone is likened to this animal; form part of lateral nasal wall

Continued

Cranial Bones and Their Markings—cont'd

Bones and Markings	Description
SPHENOID—cont'd	
Optic foramen	Opening into orbit at root of lesser wing; transmits optic nerve
Superior orbital fissure	Slitlike opening into orbit; lateral to optic foramen; transmits third, fourth, and part of fifth cranial nerves
Foramen rotundum	Opening in greater wing that transmits maxillary division of fifth cranial nerve
Foramen ovale	Opening in greater wing that transmits mandibular division of fifth cranial nerve
Foramen lacerum	Opening at the junction of the sphenoid, temporal, and occipital bones; transmits branch of the ascending pharyngeal artery
Foramen spinosum	Opening in greater wing that transmits the middle meningeal artery to supply meninges
TEMPORAL	Form lower sides of cranium and part of cranial floor; contain middle and inner ear structures
Squamous portion	Thin, flaring upper part of bone
Mastoid portion	Rough-surfaced lower part of bone posterior to external auditory meatus
Petrous portion	Wedge-shaped process that forms part of center section of cranial floor between sphenoid and occipital bones; name derived from Greek word for stone because of extreme hardness of this process; houses middle and inner ear structures
Mastoid process	Protuberance just behind ear
Mastoid air cells	Mucosa-lined, air-filled spaces within mastoid process
External auditory meatus (or canal)	Tube extending into temporal bone from external ear opening to tympanic membrane
Zygomatic process	Projection that articulates with malar (or zygomatic) bone
Internal auditory meatus	Fairly large opening on posterior surface of petrous portion of bone; transmits eighth cranial nerve to inner ear and seventh cranial nerve on its way to facial structures

Bones and Markings	Description
MANDIBULAR FOSSA	Oval-shaped depression anterior to external auditory meatus; forms for condyle of mandible
Styloid process	Slender spike of bone extending downward and forward from undersurface of bone anterior to mastoid process; often broken off in dry skull; several neck muscles and ligaments attach to styloid process
Stylomastoid foramen	Opening between styloid and mastoid processes where facial nerve emerges from cranial cavity
Jugular fossa	Depression on undersurface of petrous portion; dilated beginning of internal jugular vein lodged here
Jugular foramen	Opening in suture between petrous portion and occiptal bone; transmits lateral sinus and ninth, tenth, and eleventh cranial nerves
Carotid canal (or foramen)	Channel in perrous portion; best seen from undersurface of skull; transmits internal carotid artery
OCCIPITAL	Forms posterior part of cranial floor and walls
Foramen magnum	Hole through which spinal cord enters cranial cavity
Condyles	Convex, oval processes on either side of foramen magnum; articulate with depressions on first cervical vertebra
External occipital protuberance	Prominent projection on posterior surface in midline short distance above foramen magnum; can be felt as definite bump
Superior nuchal line	Curved ridge extending laterally from external occipital protuberance
Inferior nuchal line	Less well-defined ridge paralleling superior nuchal line a short distance below it
Internal occipital protuberance	Projection in midline on inner surface of bone; grooves for lateral sinuses extend laterally from this process and one for sagittal sinus extends upward from it

Continued

*C*ranial Bones and Their Markings—cont'd

Bones and Markings	Description
ETHMOID	Complicated irregular bone that helps make up anterior portion of cranial floor, medial wall of orbits, upper parts of nasal septum, and sidewalls and part of nasal roof; lies anterior to sphenoid and posterior to nasal bones
Horizontal (cribriform) plate	Olfactory nerves pass through numerous holes in this plate
Crista galli	Meninges (membranes around the brain) attach to this process
Perpendicular plate	Forms upper part of nasal septum
Ethmoid sinuses	Honeycombed, mucosa-lined air spaces within lateral masses of bone
Superior and middle conchae (turbinates)	Help to form lateral walls of nose
Lateral masses	Compose sides of bone; contain many air spaces (ethmoid cells or sinuses); inner surface forms superior and middle conchae

*F*acial Bones and Their Markings

Bones and Markings	Description
PALATINE	Form posterior part of hard palate, floor, and part of sidewalls of nasal cavity and floor of orbit
Horizontal plate	Joined to palatine processes of maxillae to complete part of hard palate
MANDIBLE	Lower jawbone; largest, strongest bone of face
Body	Main part of bone; forms chin
Ramus	Process, one on either side, that projects upward from posterior part of body
Condyle (or head)	Part of each ramus that articulates with mandibular fossa of temporal bone
Neck	Constricted part just below condyles
Alveolar process	Teeth set into this arch
Mandibular foramen	Opening on inner surface of ramus; transmits nerves and vessels to lower teeth
Mental foramen	Opening on outer surface below space between two bicuspids; transmits terminal branches of nerves and vessels that enter bone through mandibular foramen; dentists inject anesthetics through these foramina
Coronoid process	Projection upward from anterior part of each ramus; temporal muscle inserts here
Angle	Juncture of posterior and inferior margins of ramus
MAXILLA	Upper jaw bones; form part of floor of orbit, anterior part of roof of mouth, and floor of nose and part of sidewalls of nose
Alveolar process	Arch containing teeth
Maxillary sinus (antrum of Highmore)	Large mucosa–lined, air–filled cavity within body of each maxilla; largest of sinuses
Palatine process	Horizontal inward projection from alveolar process; forms anterior and larger part of hard palate
Infraorbital foramen	Hole on external surface just below orbit; transmits vessels and nerves

Continued

*F*acial Bones and Their Markings—cont'd

Bones and Markings	Description
MAXILLA—cont'd	
Lacrimal groove	Groove on inner surface; joined by similar groove on lacrimal bone to form canal housing nasolacrimal duct
NASAL	Small bones forming upper part of bridge of nose
ZYGOMATIC	Cheekbones; form part of floor and sidewall of orbit
LACRIMAL	Thin bones about size and shape of fingernail; posterior and lateral to nasal bones in medial wall of orbit; help form sidewall of nasal cavity, often missing in dry skull
INTERIOR NASAL CONCHAE (TURBINATES)	Thin scroll of bone forming shelf along inner surface of sidewall of nasal cavity; lies above roof of mouth
VOMER	Forms lower and posterior part of nasal septum; shaped like ploughshare

*S*pecial Features of the Skull

Feature	Description
SUTURES	Immovable joints between skull bones
Squamous	Line of articulation along top curved edge of temporal bone
Coronal	Joint between parietal bones and frontal bone
Lambdoidal	Joint between parietal bones and occipital bone
Sagittal	Joint between right and left parietal bones
FONTANELS	"Soft spots" where ossification is incomplete at birth; allow some compression of skull during birth; also important in determining position of head before delivery; six such areas located at angles of parietal bones
Frontal (or anterior)	At intersection of sagittal and coronal sutures (juncture of parietal bones and frontal bone); diamond shaped; largest of fontanels; usually closed by 1½ years of age
Occipital (or posterior)	At intersection of sagittal and lambdoidal sutures (juncture of parietal bones and occipital bone); triangular in shape; usually closed by second month
Sphenoid (or anterolateral)	At juncture of frontal, parietal, temporal, and sphenoid bones
Mastoid (or posterolateral)	At juncture of parietal, occipital, and temporal bones; usually closed by second year
AIR SINUSES	Spaces, or cavities, within bones; those that communicate with nose called *paranasal sinuses* (frontal, sphenoidal, ethmoidal, and maxillary); mastoid cells communicate with middle ear rather than nose, therefore not included among paranasal sinuses
ORBITS FORMED BY	
Frontal	Roof of orbit
Ethmoid	Medial wall
Lacrimal	Medial wall
Sphenoid	Lateral wall
Zygomatic	Lateral wall
Maxillary	Floor
Palatine	Floor

Continued

Special Features of the Skull—cont'd

Feature	Description
NASAL SEPTUM FORMED BY	Partition in midline of nasal cavity; separates cavity into right and left halves
Perpendicular plate of ethmoid bone	Forms upper part of septum
Vomer bone	Forms lower, posterior part
Cartilage	Forms anterior part
WORMIAN BONES	Small islets of bones with suture
MALLEUS, INCUS, STAPES	Tiny bones, referred to as *auditory ossicles,* in middle ear cavity in temporal bones; resemble, respectively, miniature hammer, anvil, and stirrup

The Paranasal Sinuses

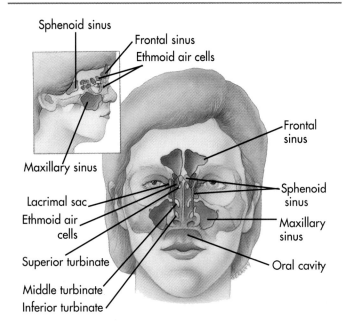

Sphenoid sinus

Frontal sinus
Ethmoid air cells

Maxillary sinus

Lacrimal sac

Ethmoid air cells

Superior turbinate

Middle turbinate

Inferior turbinate

Frontal sinus

Sphenoid sinus

Maxillary sinus

Oral cavity

The Skull at Birth

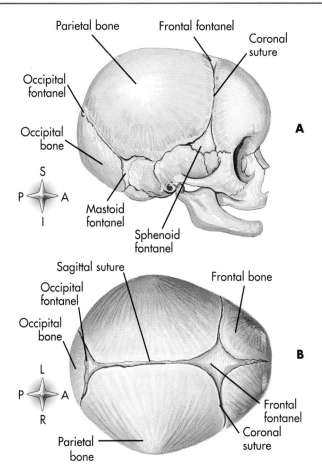

Parietal bone
Frontal fontanel
Coronal suture
Occipital fontanel
Occipital bone
Mastoid fontanel
Sphenoid fontanel

S
P — A
I

A

Sagittal suture
Occipital fontanel
Occipital bone
Frontal bone

L
P — A
R

B

Frontal fontanel
Coronal suture
Parietal bone

*H*yoid, Vertebrae, and Thoracic Bones and Their Markings

Bones and Markings	Description
HYOID	U-shaped bone in neck between mandible and upper part of larynx; distinctive as only bone in body not forming a joint with any other bone; suspended by ligaments from styloid processes of temporal bones
VERTEBRAL COLUMN	Not actually a column but a flexible, segmented curved rod; forms axis of body; head balanced above, ribs and viscera suspended in front, and lower extremities attached below; encloses spinal cord
General Features	Anterior part of each vertebra (except first two cervical) consists of body; posterior part of vertebrae consists of neural arch, which, in turn, consists of two pedicles, two laminae, and seven processes projecting from laminae
Body	Main part; flat, round mass located anteriorly; supporting or weightbearing part of vertebra
Pedicles	Short projections extending posteriorly from body
Lamina	Posterior part of vertebra to which pedicles join and from which processes project
Neural arch	Formed by pedicles and laminae; protects spinal cord posteriorly; congenital absence of one or more neural arches is known as *spina bifida* (cord may protrude right through skin)
Spinous process	Sharp process projecting inferiorly from laminae in midline
Transverse processes	Right and left lateral projections from laminae
Superior articulating processes	Project upward from laminae
Inferior articulating processes	Project downward from laminae; articulate with superior articulating processes of vertebrae below

Bones and Markings	Description
General Features—cont'd	
Spinal foramen	Hole in center of vertebra formed by union of body, pedicles, and laminae; spinal foramina, when vertebrae, superimposed one on other, form spinal cavity that houses spinal cord
Intervertebral foramina	Opening between vertebrae through which spinal nerves emerge
CERVICAL VERTEBRAE	First or upper seven vertebrae; foramen in each transverse process for transmission of vertebral artery, vein, and plexus of nerves; short bifurcated spinous processes except on seventh vertebra, where it is extra long and may be felt as protrusion when head is bent forward; bodies of these vertebrae are small, whereas spinal foramina are large and triangular
Atlas	First cervical vertebra; lacks body and spinous process; superior articulating processes are concave ovals that act as rockerlike cradles for condyles of occipital bone named *atlas* because it supports the head as Atlas supports the world in Greek mythology
Axis (epistropheus)	Second cervical vertebra, so named because atlas rotates about this bone in rotating movements of head; *dens,* or odontoid process, peglike projection upward from body of axis, forming pivot for rotation of atlas
THORACIC VERTEBRAE	Next 12 vertebrae; 12 pairs of ribs attached to these; stronger, with more massive bodies than cervical vertebrae; no transverse foramina; two sets of facets for articulations with corresponding rib: one on body, second on transverse process; upper thoracic vertebrae with elongated spinous process

Continued

Hyoid, Vertebrae, and Thoracic Bones and Their Markings—cont'd

Bones and Markings	Description
LUMBAR VERTEBRAE	Next 5 vertebrae; strong, massive; superior articulating processes directed medially instead of upward; inferior articulating processes, laterally instead of downward; short, blunt spinous process
SACRUM	Five separate vertebrae until about 25 years of age; then fused to form one wedge-shaped bone
Sacral promontory	Protuberance from anterior, upper border of sacrum into pelvis; of obstetrical importance because its size limits anteroposterior diameter of pelvic inlet
Coccyx	Four or five separate vertebrae in child but fused into one in adult
CURVES	Curves have great structural importance because they increase carrying strength of vertebral column, make balance possible in upright position (if column were straight, weight of viscera would pull body forward), absorb jolts from walking (straight column would transmit jolts straight to head), and protect column from fracture
Primary	Column curves at birth from head to sacrum with convexity posteriorly; after child stands, convexity persists only in *thoracic* and *sacral* regions, which therefore are called *primary curves*
Secondary	Concavities in *cervical* and *lumbar* regions; cervical concavity results from infant's attempts to hold head erect (2 to 4 months); lumbar concavity, from balancing efforts in learning to walk (10 to 18 months)
STERNUM	Breastbone; flat dagger-shaped bone; sternum, ribs, and thoracic vertebrae together form bony cage known as *thorax*

Bones and Markings	Description
STERNUM—cont'd	
Body	Main central part of bone
Manubrium	Flaring, upper part
Xiphoid process	Projection of cartilage at lower border of bone
RIBS	
True Ribs	Upper seven pairs; fasten to sternum by costal cartilages
False Ribs	False ribs do not attach to sternum directly; upper three pairs of false ribs attach by means of costal cartilage of seventh ribs; last two pairs do not attach to sternum at all, therefore called "floating" ribs
Head	Projection at posterior end of rib; articulates with corresponding thoracic vertebra and one above, except last three pairs, which join corresponding vertebrae only
Neck	Constricted portion just below head
Tubercle	Small knob just below neck; articulates with transverse process of corresponding thoracic vertebra; missing in lowest three ribs
Body or shaft	Main part of rib
Costal cartilage	Cartilage at sternal end of true ribs; attaches ribs (except floating ribs) to sternum

*H*yoid Bone

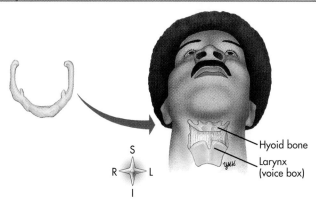

S

R ⊕ L

I

Hyoid bone

Larynx
(voice box)

Vertebral Column

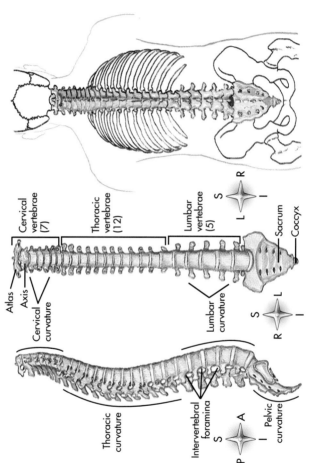

Right lateral view

Thoracic curvature

Intervertebral foramina

Pelvic curvature

S
P — A
I

Anterior view

Cervical vertebrae (7)

Thoracic vertebrae (12)

Lumbar vertebrae (5)

Atlas
Axis
Cervical curvature

Lumbar curvature

Sacrum
Coccyx

S
R — L
I

L
S — R
I

Posterior view

$\mathcal{V}$ertebrae

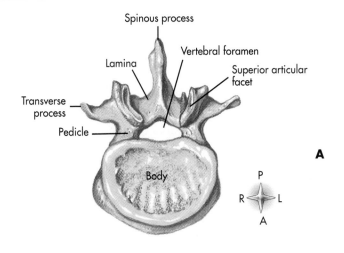

Spinous process

Lamina

Vertebral foramen

Superior articular facet

Transverse process

Pedicle

Body

A

P
R — L
A

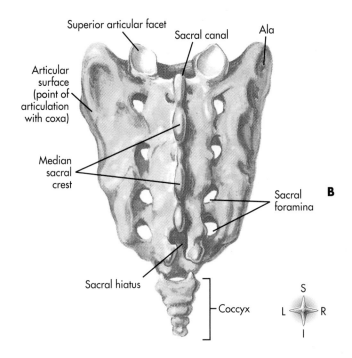

Superior articular facet

Sacral canal

Ala

Articular surface (point of articulation with coxa)

Median sacral crest

Sacral foramina

B

Sacral hiatus

Coccyx

S
L — R
I

Lumbar vertebra **(A),** superior view, and sacrum and coccyx **(B),** posterior view.

*T*horacic Cage

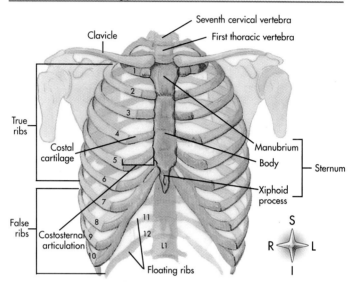

Twelve pairs of ribs, together with the vertebral column and sternum, form the bony cage known as the *thoracic cage*, or simply the *thorax*.

$\mathcal{R}$ib

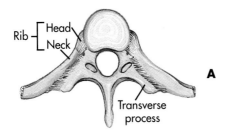

Rib $\left[\begin{array}{l}\text{Head}\\\text{Neck}\end{array}\right.$

Transverse process

A

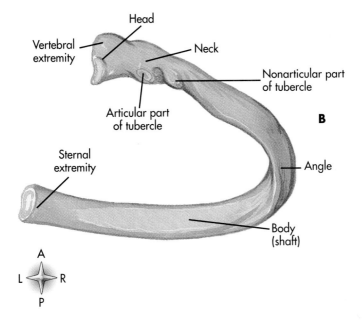

Head

Vertebral extremity

Neck

Nonarticular part of tubercle

Articular part of tubercle

B

Sternal extremity

Angle

Body (shaft)

A
L — R
P

Articulation of the ribs with the thoracic vertebra **(A)** and a rib of the left side seen from behind (posterior view) **(B).**

*U*pper Extremity Bones and Their Markings

Bones and Markings	Description
CLAVICLE	Collar bones; shoulder girdle joined to axial skeleton by articulation of clavicles with sternum (scapula does not form joint with axial skeleton)
SCAPULA	Shoulder blades; scapulae and clavicles together comprise shoulder girdle
Borders	
Superior	Upper margin
Vertebral	Margin toward vertebral column
Axillary	Lateral margin
Spine	Sharp ridge running diagonally across posterior surface of shoulder blade
Acromion process	Slightly flaring projection at lateral end of scapular spine; may be felt as tip of shoulder; articulates with clavicle
Coracoid process	Projection on anterior surface from upper border of bone; may be felt in groove between deltoid and pectoralis major muscles, about 1 inch below clavicle
Glenoid cavity	Arm socket
HUMERUS	Long bone of upper arm
Head	Smooth, hemispherical enlargement at proximal end of humerus
Anatomical neck	Oblique groove just below head
Greater tubercle	Rounded projection lateral to head on anterior surface
Lesser tubercle	Prominent projection on anterior surface just below anatomical neck
Intertubercular groove	Deep groove between greater and lesser tubercles; long tendon of biceps muscle lodges here
Surgical neck	Region just below tubercles; so named because of its liability to fracture
Deltoid tuberosity	V-shaped, rough area about midway down shaft where deltoid muscle inserts

Bones and Markings	Description
HUMERUS—cont'd	
Radial groove	Groove running obliquely downward from deltoid tuberosity; lodges radial nerve
Epicondyles (medial and lateral)	Rough projections at both sides of distal end
Capitulum	Rounded knob below lateral epicondyle; articulates with radius; sometimes called *radial* head of humerus
Trochlea	Projection with deep depression through center similar to shape of pulley; articulates with ulna
Olecranon fossa	Depression on posterior surface just above trochlea; receives olecranon process of ulna when lower arm extends
Coronoid fossa	Depression on anterior surface above trochlea; receives coronoid process of ulna in flexion of lower arm
RADIUS	Bone of thumb side of forearm
Head	Disk-shaped process forming proximal end of radius; articulates with capitulum of humerus and with radial notch of ulna
Radial tuberosity	Roughened projection on ulnar side, short distance below head; biceps muscle inserts here
Styloid process	Protuberance at distal end on lateral surface (with forearm in anatomical position)
ULNA	Bone of little finger side of forearm; longer than radius
Olecranon process	Elbow
Coronoid process	Projection on anterior surface of proximal end of ulna; trochlea of humerus fits snugly between olecranon and coronoid processes
Semilunar notch	Curved notch between olecranon and coronoid process into which trochlea fits

Continued

*U*pper Extremity Bones and Their Markings—cont'd

Bones and Markings	Description
ULNA—cont'd	
Radial notch	Curved notch lateral and inferior to semilunar notch; head of radius fits into this concavity
Head	Rounded process at distal end; does not articulate with wrist bones but with fibro-cartilaginous disk
Styloid process	Sharp protuberance at distal end; can be seen from outside on posterior surface
CARPALS	Wrist bones; arranged in two rows at proximal end of hand; proximal row (from little finger toward thumb)—*pisiform, triquetrum, lunate,* and *scaphoid;* distal row—*hamate, capitate, trapezoid,* and *trapezium*
METACARPALS	Long bones forming framework of palm of hand; numbered I through V
PHALANGES	Miniature long bones of fingers, three (proximal, middle, distal) in each finger, two (proximal, distal) in each thumb

Right Scapula

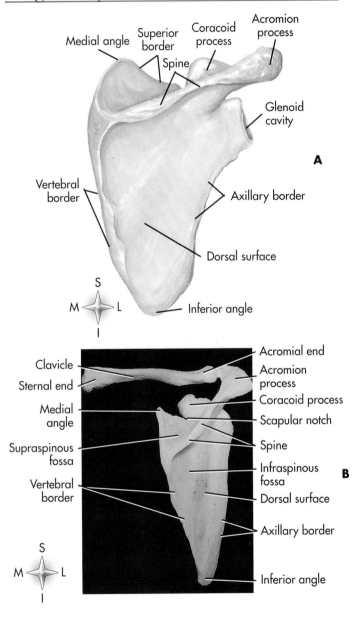

Posterior view of scapula only **(A)** and posterior view showing articulation of the scapula with the clavicle **(B)**.

Bones of the Arm (Anterior View)

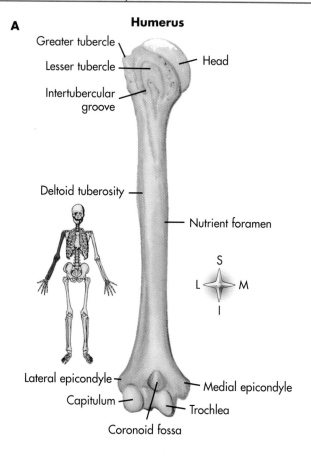

A

Humerus

Greater tubercle
Lesser tubercle
Intertubercular groove
Head

Deltoid tuberosity

Nutrient foramen

S
L ◇ M
I

Lateral epicondyle
Capitulum
Medial epicondyle
Trochlea
Coronoid fossa

A, Humerus (upper arm). (The *inset* shows the relative position of the right arm bones within the entire skeleton.)

Right Scapula

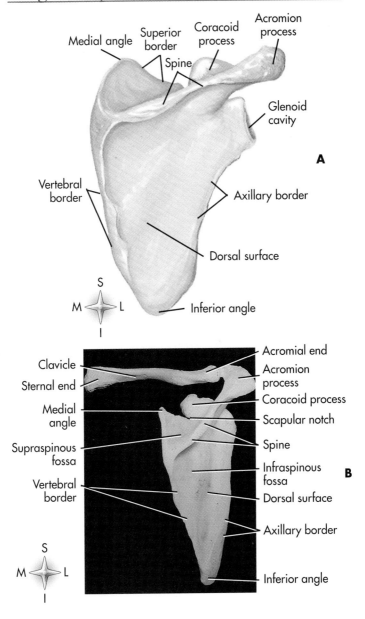

Posterior view of scapula only **(A)** and posterior view showing articulation of the scapula with the clavicle **(B).**

ℬones of the Arm (Anterior View)

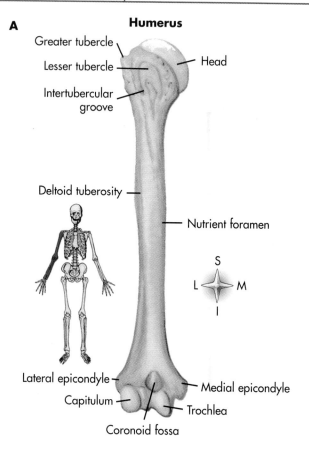

A, Humerus (upper arm). (The *inset* shows the relative position of the right arm bones within the entire skeleton.)

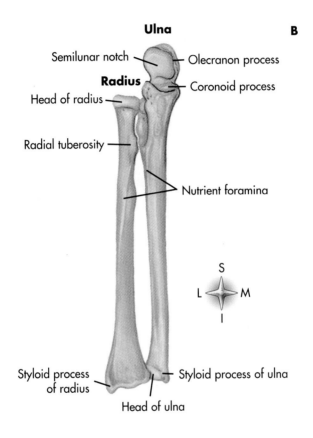

B, Radius and ulna (forearm).   *Continued*

*B*ones of the Arm (Anterior View)—cont'd

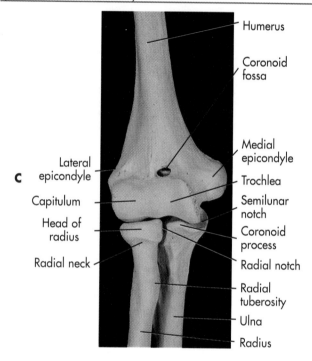

Humerus

Coronoid fossa

Medial epicondyle

Trochlea

Semilunar notch

Coronoid process

Radial notch

Radial tuberosity

Ulna

Radius

Lateral epicondyle

C

Capitulum

Head of radius

Radial neck

C, Elbow joint, showing how the distal end of the humerus joins the proximal ends of the radius and ulna.

$\mathscr{B}$ones of the Arm (Posterior View)

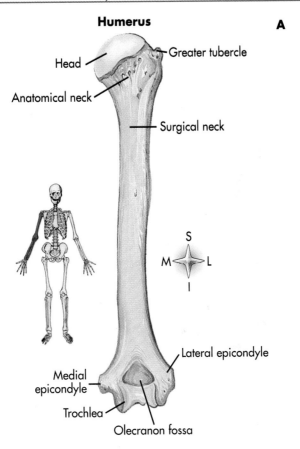

Humerus

A

Greater tubercle

Head

Anatomical neck

Surgical neck

S

M — L

I

Lateral epicondyle

Medial epicondyle

Trochlea

Olecranon fossa

A, Humerus (upper arm). (The *inset* shows the relative position of the right arm within the entire skeleton.) *Continued*

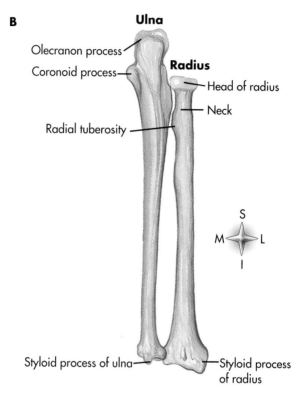

B, Radius and ulna (forearm).

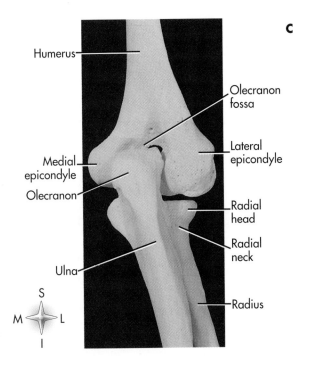

C, Elbow joint, showing how the distal end of the humerus joins the proximal ends of the radius and ulna.

ℬones of the Hand and Wrist

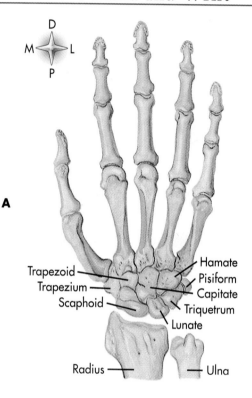

A, Dorsal view of the right hand and wrist.

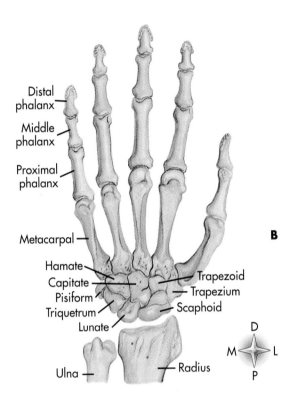

Distal phalanx

Middle phalanx

Proximal phalanx

Metacarpal

Hamate

Capitate

Pisiform

Triquetrum

Lunate

Trapezoid

Trapezium

Scaphoid

Ulna

Radius

B

D

M — L

P

B, Palmar view of the right hand and wrist.

*L*ower Extremity Bones and Their Markings

Bones and Markings	Description
Coxal	Large hip bone; with sacrum and coccyx, forms basinlike pelvic cavity; lower extremities attached to axial skeleton by coxal bones
Ilium	Upper, flaring portion
Ischium	Lower, posterior portion
Pubic bone (pubis)	Medial, anterior section
Acetabulum	Hip socket; formed by union of ilium, ischium, and pubis
Iliac crests	Upper, curving boundary of ilium
Iliac spines	
Anterior superior	Prominent projection at anterior end of iliac crest; can be felt externally as "point" of hip
Anterior inferior	Less prominent projection short distance below anterior superior spine
Posterior superior	At posterior end of iliac crest
Posterior inferior	Just below posterior superior spine
Greater sciatic notch	Large notch on posterior surface of ilium just below posterior inferior spine
Ischial tuberosity	Large, rough, quadrilateral process forming inferior part of ischium; in erect sitting position body rests on these tuberosities
Ischial spine	Pointed projection just above tuberosity
Symphysis pubis	Cartilaginous, amphiarthrotic joint between pubic bones
Superior ramus of pubis	Part of pubis lying between symphysis and acetabulum; forms upper part of obturator foramen
Inferior ramus	Part extending down from symphysis; unites with ischium
Pubic arch	Angle formed by two inferior rami
Pubic crest	Upper margin of superior ramus
Pubic tubercle	Rounded process at end of crest
Obturator foramen	Large hole in anterior surface of os coxa; formed by pubis and ischium; largest foramen in body

Bones and Markings	Description
Pelvic brim (or inlet)	Boundary of aperture leading into true pelvis; formed by pubic crests, iliopectineal lines, and sacral promontory; size and shape of this inlet have obstetrical importance, because if any of its diameters are too small, infant skull cannot enter true pelvis for natural birth
True pelvis (or pelvis minor)	Space below pelvic brim; true "basin" with bone and muscle walls and muscle floor; pelvic organs located in this space
False pelvis (or pelvis major)	Broad, shallow space above pelvic brim, or pelvic inlet; name "false pelvis" is misleading, because this space is actually part of abdominal cavity, not pelvic cavity
Pelvic outlet	Irregular circumference marking lower limits of true pelvis; bounded by tip of coccyx and two ischial tuberosities
Pelvic girdle (or bony pelvis)	Complete bony ring; composed of two hip bones (ossa coxae), sacrum, and coccyx; forms firm base by which trunk rests on thighs and for attachment of lower extremities to axial skeleton
FEMUR	Thigh bone; largest, strongest bone of body
Head	Rounded, upper end of bone; fits into acetabulum
Neck	Constricted portion just below head
Greater trochanter	Protuberance located inferiorly and laterally to head
Lesser trochanter	Small protuberance located inferiorly and medially to greater trochanter
Intertrochanteric line	Line extending between greater and lesser trochanter
Linea aspera	Prominent ridge extending lengthwise along concave posterior surface
Supracondylar ridges	Two ridges formed by division of linea aspera at its lower end; medial supracondylar ridge extends inward to inner condyle, lateral ridge to outer condyle

Continued

*L*ower Extremity Bones and Their Markings—cont'd

Bones and Markings	Description
FEMUR—cont'd	
Condyles	Large, rounded bulges at distal end of femur; one medial and one lateral
Epicondyles	Blunt projections from the sides of the condyles; one on the medial aspect and one on the lateral aspect
Adductor tubercle	Small projection just above medial condyle; marks termination of medial supracondylar ridge
Trochlea	Smooth depression between condyles on anterior surface; articulates with patella
Intercondyloid fossa (notch)	Deep depression between condyles on posterior surface; cruciate ligaments that help bind femur to tibia lodge in this notch
PATELLA	Kneecap; largest sesamoid bone of body; embedded in tendon of quadriceps femoris muscle
TIBIA	Shin bone
Condyles	Bulging prominences at proximal end of tibia; upper surfaces concave for articulation with femur
Intercondylar eminence	Upward projection on articular surface between condyles
Crest	Sharp ridge on anterior surface
Tibial tuberosity	Projection in midline on anterior surface
Medial malleolus	Rounded downward projection at distal end of tibia; forms prominence on medial surface of ankle

Bones and Markings	Description
FIBULA	Long, slender bone of lateral side of lower leg
Lateral malleolus	Rounded prominence at distal end of fibula; forms prominence on lateral surface of ankle
TARSALS	Bones that form heel and proximal or posterior half of foot
Calcaneus	Heel bone
Talus	Uppermost of tarsals; articulates with tibia and fibula; boxed in by medial and lateral malleoli
Longitudinal arches	Tarsals and metatarsals so arranged as to form arch from front to back of foot
Medial	Formed by calcaneus, talus, navicular, cuneiforms, and three medial metatarsals
Lateral	Formed by calcaneus, cuboid, and two lateral metatarsals
Transverse (or metatarsal) arch	Metatarsals and distal row of tarsals (cuneiforms and cuboid) so articulated as to form arch across foot; bones kept in two arched positions by means of powerful ligaments in sole of foot and by muscles and tendons
METATARSALS	Long bones of feet
PHALANGES	Miniature long bones of toes; two in each great toe; three in other toes

The Female Pelvis

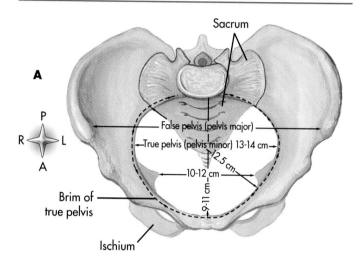

A, Pelvis viewed from above. Note that the brim of the true pelvis (*dotted line*) marks the boundary between the superior false pelvis (*pelvis major*) and the inferior true pelvis (*pelvis minor*). B, Pelvis viewed from below.

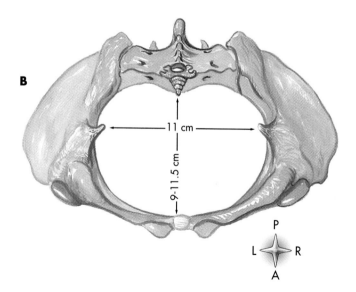

$\mathscr{R}$ight Coxal Bone

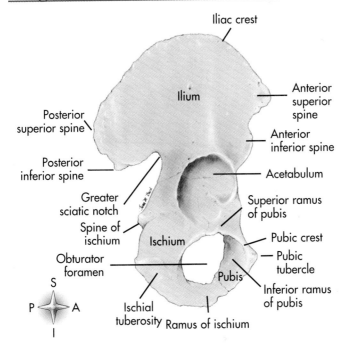

Iliac crest

Ilium

Posterior superior spine

Anterior superior spine

Anterior inferior spine

Posterior inferior spine

Acetabulum

Greater sciatic notch

Superior ramus of pubis

Spine of ischium

Ischium

Pubic crest

Obturator foramen

Pubic tubercle

Pubis

S

Inferior ramus of pubis

P A

Ischial tuberosity

Ramus of ischium

I

The right coxal bone is disarticulated from the skeleton and viewed from the side with the bone turned so as to look directly into the acetabulum.

*B*ones of the Thigh and Leg

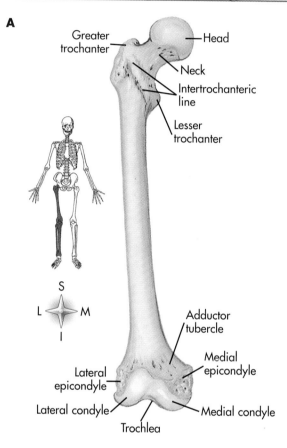

A, Right femur, anterior surface.

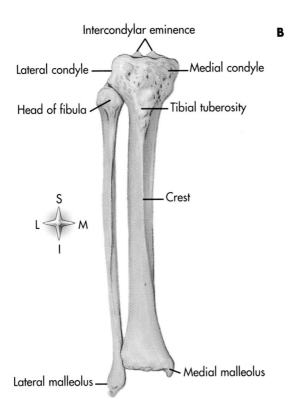

B, Right tibia and fibula, anterior surface. (The *inset* [p. 156] shows the relative position of the bones of the thigh and leg within the entire skeleton.)

*B*ones of the Foot

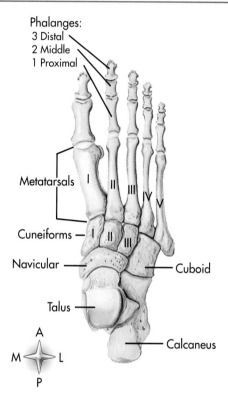

Phalanges:
3 Distal
2 Middle
1 Proximal

Metatarsals

I
II
III
IV
V

Cuneiforms — I
II
III

Navicular

Cuboid

Talus

Calcaneus

A
M ◄►► L
P

Bones of the right foot viewed from above. Tarsal bones consist of cuneiforms, navicular, talus, cuboid, and calcaneus.

Arches of the Foot

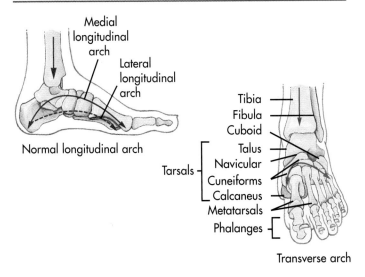

Transverse arch

The medial portion of the longitudinal arch is formed by calcaneus, cuboid, and two lateral metatarsals. The transverse arch is in the metatarsal region of the right foot.

Comparison of Male and Female Skeletons

Portion of Skeleton	Male	Female
GENERAL FORM	Bones heavier and thicker	Bones lighter and thinner
	Muscle attachment sites more massive	Muscle attachment sites less distinct
	Joint surfaces relatively large	Joint surfaces relatively small
SKULL	Forehead shorter vertically	Forehead more elongated vertically
	Mandible and maxillae relatively larger	Mandible and maxillae relatively smaller
	Facial area more pronounced	Facial area rounder, with less pronounced features
	Processes more prominent	Processes less pronounced
PELVIS		
Pelvic cavity	Narrower in all dimensions	Wider in all dimensions
	Deeper	Shorter and roomier
	Pelvic outlet relatively small	Pelvic outlet relatively large
Sacrum	Long, narrow, with smooth concavity (sacral curvature); sacral promontory more pronounced	Short, wide, flat concavity more pronounced in a posterior direction; sacral promontory less pronounced
Coccyx	Less movable	More movable and follows posterior direction of sacral curvature
Pubic arch	Less than a 90-degree angle	Greater than a 90-degree angle
Symphysis pubis	Relatively deep	Relatively shallow
Ischial spine, ischial tuberosity, and anterior superior iliac spine	Turned more inward	Turned more outward and further apart
Greater sciatic notch	Narrow	Wide

*C*omparison of the Male and Female Bony Pelvis

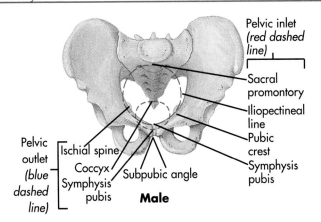

Pelvic inlet
(red dashed line)

Sacral promontory

Iliopectineal line

Pubic crest

Symphysis pubis

Pelvic outlet (blue dashed line)

Ischial spine

Coccyx

Symphysis pubis

Subpubic angle

Male

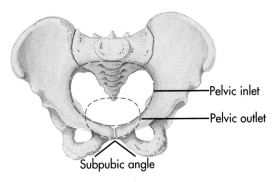

Pelvic inlet

Pelvic outlet

Subpubic angle

Female

Classification of Fibrous and Cartilaginous Joints

Types	Examples	Structural Features	Movements
FIBROUS JOINTS			
Syndesmoses	Joints between distal ends of radius and ulna	Fibrous bands (ligaments) connect articulating bones	Slight
Sutures	Joints between skull bones	Teethlike projections of articulating bones interlock with thin layer of fibrous tissue connecting them	None
Gomphoses	Joints between roots of teeth and jaw bones	Fibrous tissue connects roots of teeth to alveolar processes	None
CARTILAGINOUS JOINTS			
Synchondroses	Costal cartilage attachments of first rib to sternum; epiphyseal plate between diaphysis and epiphysis of growing long bone	Hyaline cartilage connects articulating bones	Slight
Symphyses	Symphysis pubis; joints between *bodies of vertebrae*	Fibrocartilage between articulating bones	Slight

Structure of Synovial Joints

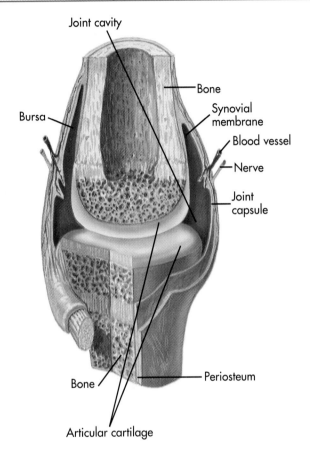

Joint cavity

Bone

Bursa

Synovial membrane

Blood vessel

Nerve

Joint capsule

Bone

Periosteum

Articular cartilage

Synovial Joint Types

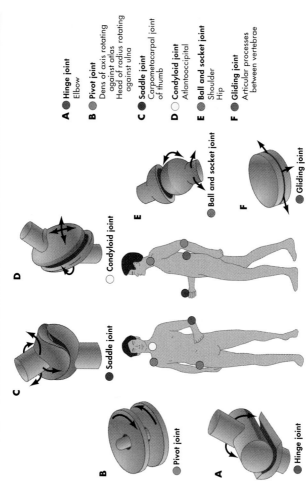

A ● **Hinge joint**
Elbow

B ● **Pivot joint**
Dens of axis rotating
against atlas
Head of radius rotating
against ulna

C ● **Saddle joint**
Carpometacarpal joint
of thumb

D ○ **Condyloid joint**
Atlantooccipital

E ● **Ball and socket joint**
Shoulder
Hip

F ● **Gliding joint**
Articular processes
between vertebrae

Uniaxial: **A**, hinge and, **B**, pivot. *Biaxial:* **C**, saddle and, **D**, condyloid. *Multiaxial:* **E**, ball and socket; and, **F**, gliding.

Classification of Synovial Joints

Types	Examples	Type	Movements
UNIAXIAL			
Hinge	Elbow joint	Spool-shaped process fits into concave socket	Around one axis; in one plane Flexion and extension only
Pivot	Joint between first and second cervical vertebrae	Arch-shaped process fits around peglike process	Rotation
BIAXIAL			Around two axes, perpendicular to each other; in two planes
Saddle	Thumb joint between first metacarpal and carpal bone	Saddle-shaped bone fits into socket that is concave–convex–concave	Flexion, extension in one plane; abduction; adduction in other plane; opposing thumb to fingers
Condyloid (ellipsoidal)	Joint between radius and carpal bones	Oval condyle fits into elliptical socket	Flexion, extension in one plane; abduction, adduction in other plane
MULTIAXIAL			Around many axes
Ball and socket	Shoulder joint and hip joint	Ball-shaped process fits into concave socket	Widest range of movements; flexion, extension, abduction, adduction, rotation, circumduction
Gliding	Joints between articular facets of adjacent vertebrae; joints between carpal and tarsal bones	Relatively flat articulating surfaces	Gliding movements without any angular or circular movements

*S*houlder Joint

A

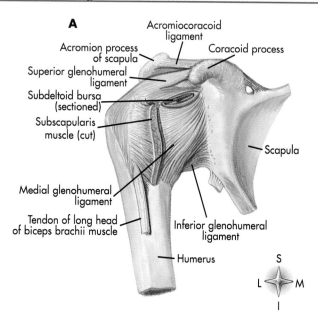

Acromiocoracoid ligament

Acromion process of scapula

Coracoid process

Superior glenohumeral ligament

Subdeltoid bursa (sectioned)

Subscapularis muscle (cut)

Scapula

Medial glenohumeral ligament

Tendon of long head of biceps brachii muscle

Inferior glenohumeral ligament

Humerus

S
L M
I

B

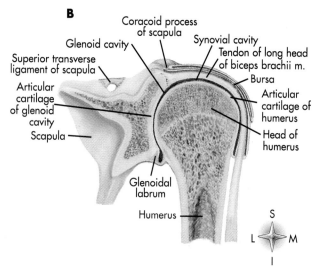

Coracoid process of scapula

Glenoid cavity

Synovial cavity

Superior transverse ligament of scapula

Tendon of long head of biceps brachii m.

Articular cartilage of glenoid cavity

Bursa

Scapula

Articular cartilage of humerus

Head of humerus

Glenoidal labrum

Humerus

S
L M
I

A, Anterior view of the shoulder joint. **B,** Shoulder joint viewed from behind through the shoulder joint.

*H*ip Joint

A

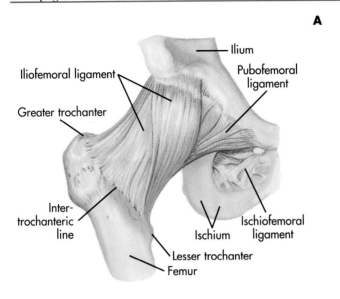

Iliofemoral ligament

Greater trochanter

Ilium

Pubofemoral ligament

Inter-trochanteric line

Ischium

Ischiofemoral ligament

Lesser trochanter

Femur

B

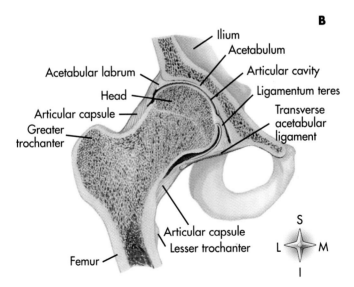

Acetabular labrum

Head

Articular capsule

Greater trochanter

Ilium

Acetabulum

Articular cavity

Ligamentum teres

Transverse acetabular ligament

Articular capsule

Lesser trochanter

Femur

S
L ✦ M
I

A, Anterior view of the hip joint. **B,** Frontal section through the hip joint.

$\mathscr{R}$ight Knee Joint

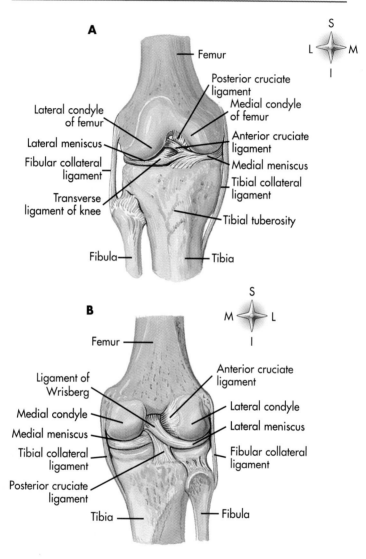

A, Viewed from in front. **B,** Viewed from behind.

Sagittal Section Through Knee Joint

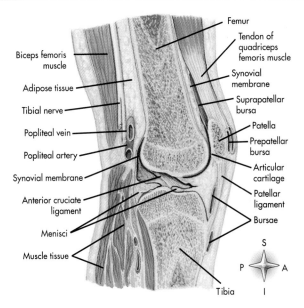

Femur

Tendon of quadriceps femoris muscle

Biceps femoris muscle

Synovial membrane

Adipose tissue

Suprapatellar bursa

Tibial nerve

Patella

Popliteal vein

Prepatellar bursa

Popliteal artery

Articular cartilage

Synovial membrane

Patellar ligament

Anterior cruciate ligament

Bursae

Menisci

Muscle tissue

Tibia

S
P — A
I

Vertebrae and Their Ligaments

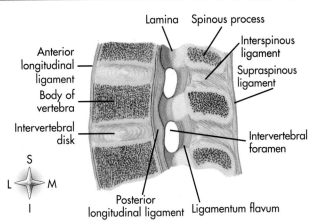

Lamina   Spinous process

Anterior longitudinal ligament

Interspinous ligament

Supraspinous ligament

Body of vertebra

Intervertebral disk

Intervertebral foramen

S
L — M
I

Posterior longitudinal ligament   Ligamentum flavum

This sagittal section shows two lumbar vertebrae and their ligaments.

$\mathscr{S}$ynovial (Diarthrotic) and Two Cartilaginous (Amphiarthrotic) Joints

Name	Articulating Bones	Type	Movements
Atlantoepistropheal	Anterior arch of atlas rotates about dens of axis (epistropheus)	Synovial (pivot)	Pivoting or partial rotation of head
Vertebral	Between bodies of vertebrae	Cartilaginous (symphyses)	Slight movement between any two vertebrae but considerable motility for column as whole
Sternoclavicular	Between articular processes	Synovial (gliding)	Gliding
	Medial end of clavicle with manubrium of sternum	Synovial (gliding)	Gliding
Acromioclavicular	Distal end of clavicle with acromion of scapula	Synovial (gliding)	Gliding; elevation, depression, protraction, and retraction
Thoracic	Heads of ribs with bodies of vertebrae	Synovial (gliding)	Gliding
	Tubercles of ribs with transverse processes of vertebrae	Synovial (gliding)	Gliding
Shoulder	Head of humerus in glenoid cavity of scapula	Synovial (ball and socket)	Flexion, extension, abduction, adduction, rotation, and circumduction of upper arm

Joint	Articulation	Type	Movement
Elbow	Trochlea of humerus with semilunar notch of ulna; head of radius with capitulum of humerus	Synovial (hinge)	Flexion and extension
	Head of radius in radial notch of ulna	Synovial (pivot)	Supination and pronation of lower arm and hand; rotation of lower arm on upper extremity
Wrist	Scaphoid, lunate, and triquetral bones articulate with radius and articular disk	Synovial (condyloid)	Flexion, extension, abduction, and adduction of hand
Carpal	Between various carpals	Synovial (gliding)	Gliding
Hand	Proximal end of first metacarpal with trapezium	Synovial (saddle)	Flexion, extension, abduction, adduction, and circumduction of thumb and opposition to fingers
	Distal end of metacarpals with proximal end of phalanges	Synovial (hinge)	Flexion, extension, limited abduction, and adduction of fingers
	Between phalanges	Synovial (hinge)	Flexion and extension of finger sections
Sacroiliac	Between sacrum and two ilia	Synovial (gliding)	None or slight

Synovial (Diarthrotic) and Two Cartilaginous (Amphiarthrotic) Joints—cont'd

Name	Articulating Bones	Type	Movements
Symphysis pubis	Between two pubic bones	Cartilaginous (symphysis)	Slight, particularly during pregnancy and delivery
Hip	Head of femur in acetabulum of os coxae	Synovial (ball and socket)	Flexion, extension, abduction, adduction, rotation, and circumduction
Knee	Between distal end of femur and proximal end of tibia	Synovial (hinge)	Flexion and extension; slight rotation of tibia
Tibiofibular (proximal)	Head of fibula with lateral condyle of tibia	Synovial (gliding)	Gliding
Ankle	Distal ends of tibia and fibula with talus	Synovial (hinge)	Flexion (dorsiflexion) and extension (plantar flexion)
Foot	Between tarsals	Synovial (gliding)	Gliding; inversion and eversion
	Between metatarsals and phalanges	Synovial (hinge)	Flexion, extension, slight abduction, and adduction
	Between phalanges	Synovial (hinge)	Flexion and extension

Types of Joint Movements

Term	Description
Flexion	Decreases the angle between bones as when the head is bent forward to the chest
Extension	Increases the angle between bones; returns a part from its flexed position to its anatomical position
Rotation	Consists of pivoting a bone on its own axis as when moving the head from side to side to indicate "no"
Hyperextension	Stretching an extended part beyond its anatomical position as the arms in preparation to do a standing broad jump
Abduction	Moves a part away from the median plane of the body as when moving the legs out to the side in performing a "jumping jack"
Adduction	Moves a part toward the median plane of the body
Supination	Rotation of the forearm and hand so that the palm faces forward or upward and the radius lies parallel to the ulna; a corresponding movement can be made with the leg and foot
Pronation	Rotation of the hand and forearm so the palm faces backward or downward
Dorsiflexion	A movement in which the top of the foot is elevated (brought toward the front of the lower leg) with toes pointing upward
Plantar flexion	A movement in which the bottom of the foot is directed downward; this motion allows a person to stand on tiptoe
Inversion	Turning the sole of the foot inward; this movement rolls the big toe of the foot upward and away from the body
Eversion	Turning the arch side of the foot downward; this movement rolls the little toe of the foot upward and toward the body
Retraction	Moving a part inward toward the body as when the jaw is pulled back
Protraction	Moving a part away from the body as when the jaw is thrust forward
Elevation	Moves a part up as in closing the mouth
Depression	Lowers a part as in opening the mouth, thereby lowering the jaw

Muscular System

There are over 600 skeletal muscles in the human body. Collectively, they constitute 40% to 50% of a person's body weight. And, together with the scaffolding provided by the skeleton, muscles also determine the form and contours of the body.

General Overview of the Body Musculature

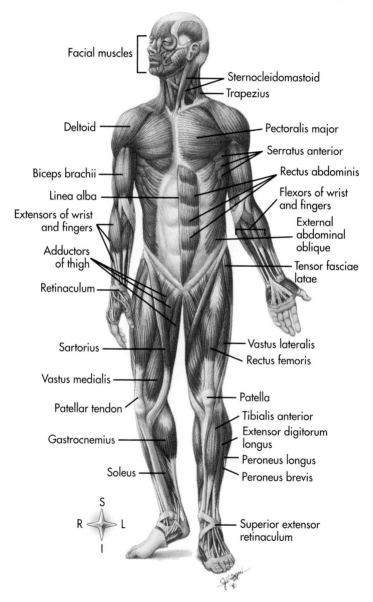

Facial muscles
Sternocleidomastoid
Trapezius
Deltoid
Pectoralis major
Serratus anterior
Biceps brachii
Rectus abdominis
Linea alba
Flexors of wrist and fingers
Extensors of wrist and fingers
External abdominal oblique
Adductors of thigh
Retinaculum
Tensor fasciae latae
Sartorius
Vastus lateralis
Rectus femoris
Vastus medialis
Patella
Patellar tendon
Tibialis anterior
Extensor digitorum longus
Gastrocnemius
Peroneus longus
Soleus
Peroneus brevis
Superior extensor retinaculum

S
R — L
I

Anterior view of the body musculature.

General Overview of the Body Musculature—cont'd

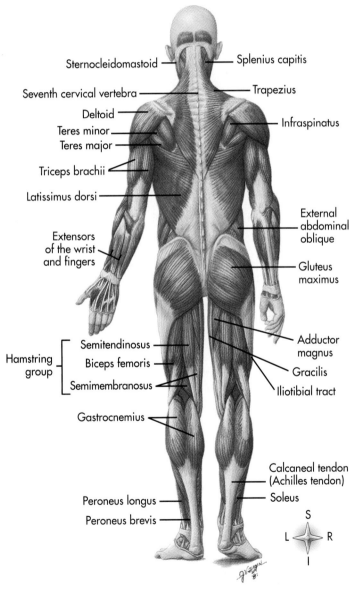

Posterior view of the body musculature.

*S*tructure of Skeletal Muscle

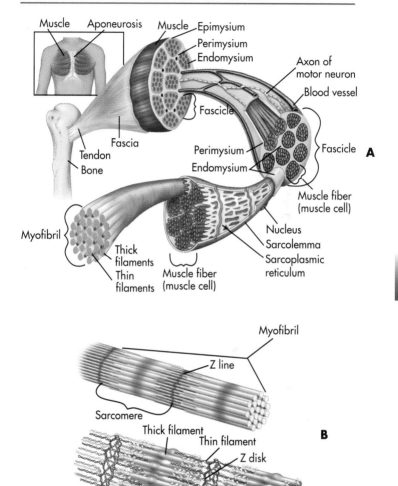

Note in *part A* of the illustration above that the connective tissue covers the epimysium, perimysium, and endomysium are continuous with each other and with the tendon. The muscle fibers are held together by the perimysium in groups called *fascicles*. The magnification of the myofibril, *part B*, further shows sarcomere between successive Z lines (Z disks). Cross striae are visible. The molecular structure of myofibril shows thick myofilaments and thin myofilaments.

Sarcomere

Sarcomere is the basic contractile unit of the muscle cell.

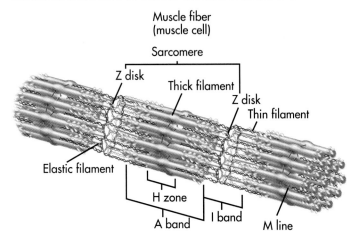

Z line: A dense plate or disk to which the thin filaments directly anchor. Also called *Z disk*.

M line: Protein molecules that hold the thick (myosin) filaments together.

A band: The segment that runs the entire length of the thick filaments.

I band: The segment that includes the Z line (disk) and the ends of the thin filaments where they do not overlap the thick filaments.

H zone: The middle region of the thick filaments where they do not overlap the thin filaments.

𝒰nique Features of the Skeletal Muscle Cell

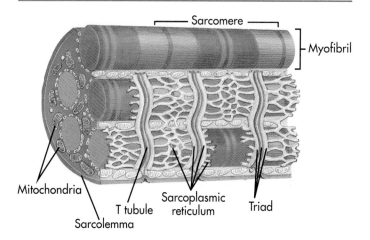

The *T tubules* are extensions of the plasma membrane, or *sarcolemna*. The *sarcoplasmic reticulum* forms the network of tubular canals and sacs. A *triad* is a triplet of adjacent tubules: a terminal (end) sac of the sarcoplasmic reticulum, a T tubule, and another terminal sac of the sarcoplasmic reticulum.

Structure of Myofilaments

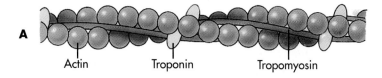

A   Actin   Troponin   Tropomyosin

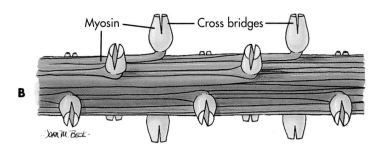

B   Myosin — Cross bridges —

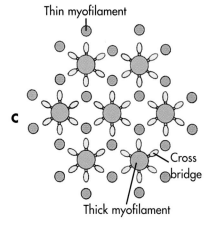

C   Thin myofilament   Cross bridge   Thick myofilament

This illustration depicts, **A,** thin myofilament, **B,** thick myofilament, and, **C,** a cross section of several thick and thin myofilaments, showing the relative positions of myofilaments and cross bridges.

*M*ajor Events of Muscle Contraction and Relaxation

Excitation and contraction

1. A nerve impulse reaches the end of a motor neuron, triggering the release of the neurotransmitter *acetylcholine.*

2. Acetylcholine diffuses rapidly across the gap of the neuromuscular junction and binds to acetylcholine receptors on the motor endplate of the muscle fiber.

3. Stimulation of acetylcholine receptors initiates an impulse that travels along the sarcolemma, through the T tubules, to sacs of the sarcoplasmic reticulum.

4. Ca^{++} is released from the sarcoplasmic reticulum into the sarcoplasm, where it binds to troponin molecules in the thin myofilaments.

5. Tropomyosin molecules in the thin myofilaments shift, exposing actin's active sites.

6. Energized myosin cross bridges of the thick myofilaments bind to actin and use their energy to pull the thin myofilaments toward the center of each sarcomere. This cycle repeats itself many times per second, as long as adenosine triphosphate (ATP) is available.

7. As the thin filaments slide past the thick myofilaments, the entire muscle fiber shortens.

Relaxation

1. After the impulse is over, the sarcoplasmic reticulum begins actively pumping Ca^{++} back into its sacs.

2. As Ca^{++} is stripped from troponin molecules in the thin myofilaments, tropomyosin returns to its position, blocking actin's active sites.

3. Myosin cross bridges are prevented from binding to actin and thus can no longer sustain the contraction.

4. Since the thick and thin myofilaments are no longer connected, the muscle fiber may return to its longer, resting length.

Effects of Excitation on a Muscle Fiber

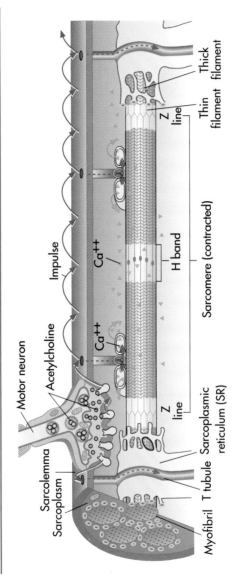

Excitation of the sarcolemma by a nerve impulse initiates an impulse in the sarcolemma. The impulse travels across the sarcolemma and through the T tubules, where it triggers adjacent sacs of the sarcoplasmic reticulum to release a flood of calcium ions (Ca^{++}) into the sarcoplasm. The Ca^{++} are then free to bind to troponin molecules in the thin filaments. This binding, in turn, initiates the chemical reactions that produce a contraction.

Molecular Basis of Muscle Contraction

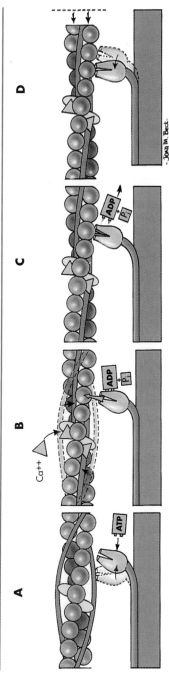

A, Each myosin cross bridge in the thick filament moves into a resting position after an ATP binds and transfers its energy. **B,** Calcium ions released from the sarcoplasmic reticulum bind to troponin in the thin filament, allowing tropomyosin to shift from its position blocking the active sites of actin molecules. **C,** Each myosin cross bridge then binds to an active site on a thin filament, displacing the remnants of ATP hydrolysis—adenosine diphosphate (ADP) and inorganic phosphate (P₁). **D,** The release of stored energy from step **A** provides the force needed for each cross bridge to move back to its original position, pulling actin along with it. Each cross bridge will remain bound to actin until another ATP binds to it and pulls it back into its resting position **(A).**

Sliding Filament Theory

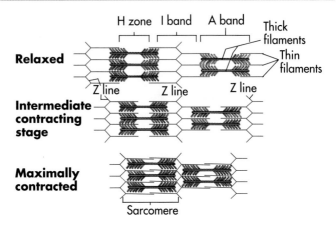

During contraction, myosin cross bridges pull the thin filaments toward the center of each sarcomere, thus shortening the myofibril and the entire muscle fiber.

$\mathscr{M}$yograms of Various Types of Muscle Contractions

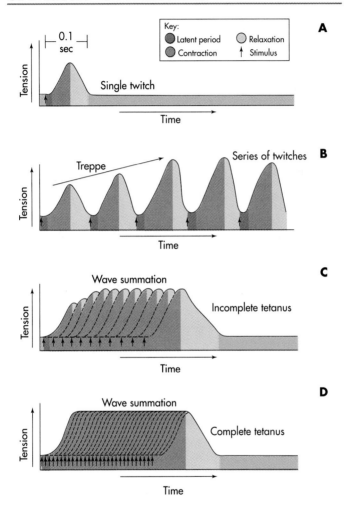

A, A single twitch contraction. **B,** The treppe phenomenon, or "staircase effect," is a steplike increase in the force of contraction over the first few in a series of twitches. **C,** Incomplete tetanus occurs when a rapid succession of stimuli produces "twitches" that seem to add together (wave summation) to produce a rather sustained contraction. **D,** Complete tetanus is a smoother sustained contraction, produced by the summation of "twitches" that occur so close together that the muscle cannot relax at all.

Characteristics of Muscle Tissues

	Skeletal	Cardiac	Smooth
PRINCIPAL LOCATION	Skeletal muscle organs	Wall of heart	Walls of many hollow organs
PRINCIPAL FUNCTIONS	Movement of bones, heat production, posture	Pumping of blood	Movement in walls of hollow organs (peristalsis, mixing)
TYPE OF CONTROL	Voluntary	Involuntary	Involuntary
STRUCTURAL FEATURES			
Striations	Present	Present	Absent
Nucleus	Many near sarcolemma	Single	Single; near center of cell
T tubules	Narrow; form triads with SR	Large diameter; form diads with SR, regulate Ca^{++} entry into sarcoplasm	Absent
Sarcoplasmic reticulum	Extensive; stores and releases Ca^{++}	Less extensive than in skeletal muscle	Very poorly developed
Cell junctions	No gap junctions	Intercalated disks	Visceral: many gap junctions Multiunit: few gap junctions
CONTRACTION STYLE	Rapid twitch contractions of motor units usually summate to produce sustained tetanic contractions; must be stimulated by a neuron	Syncytium of fibers compress heart chambers in slow, separate contractions (does not exhibit tetanus or fatigue); exhibits autorhythmicity	Visceral: electrically coupled sheets of fibers contract autorhythmically, producing peristalsis or mixing movements Multiunit: individual fibers contract when stimulated by neuron

Cardiac Muscle Fiber

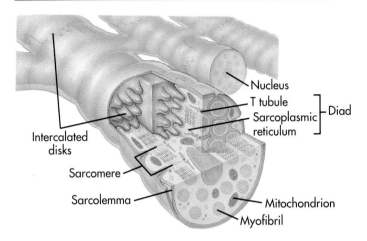

Nucleus
T tubule
Sarcoplasmic ⎤ Diad
reticulum ⎦
Intercalated
disks
Sarcomere
Sarcolemma
Mitochondrion
Myofibril

Unlike other types of muscle fibers, the cardiac muscle fiber is typically branched and forms junctions, called *intercalated disks,* with adjacent cardiac muscle fibers. Like skeletal muscle fibers, cardiac muscle fibers contain sarcoplasmic reticula and T tubules—although these structures are not as highly organized as in skeletal muscle fibers.

*S*mooth Muscle Fiber

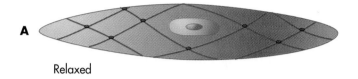

A

Relaxed

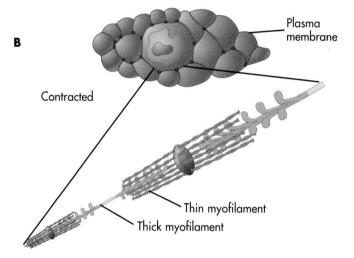

B

Plasma
membrane

Contracted

Thin myofilament

Thick myofilament

A, Thin bundles of myofilaments span the diameter of a relaxed fiber. **B,** During contraction, sliding of the myofilaments causes the fiber to shorten by "balling up." The figure shows that the fiber becomes shorter and thicker, exhibiting "dimples" where the myofilament bundles are pulling on the plasma membrane.

Attachment of a Skeletal Muscle

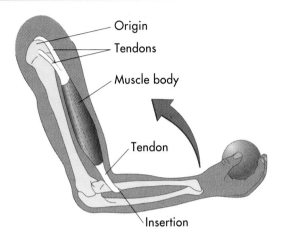

Origin

Tendons

Muscle body

Tendon

Insertion

A muscle originates at a relatively stable part of the skeleton (*origin*) and inserts at the skeletal part that is moved when the muscle contracts (*insertion*).

ℐelected Muscles Grouped According to Location

Location	Muscles
Neck	Sternocleidomastoid
Back	Trapezius
	Latissimus dorsi
Chest	Pectoralis major
	Serratus anterior
Abdominal wall	External oblique
Shoulder	Deltoid
Upper arm	Biceps brachii
	Triceps brachii
	Brachialis
Forearm	Brachioradialis
	Pronator teres
Buttocks	Gluteus maximus
	Gluteus minimus
	Gluteus medius
	Tensor fascia latae
Thigh	
Anterior surface	Quadriceps femoris group
	Rectus femoris
	Vastus lateralis
	Vastus medialis
	Vastus intermedius
Medial surface	Gracilis
	Adductor group (brevis, longus, magnus)
Posterior surface	Hamstring group
	Biceps femoris
	Semitendinosus
	Semimembranosus
Leg	
Anterior surface	Tibialis anterior
Posterior surface	Gastrocnemius
	Soleus
Pelvic floor	Levator ani
	Levator coccygeus
	Rectococcygeus

Selected Muscles Grouped According to Function

Part Moved	Example of Flexor	Example of Extensor	Example of Abductor	Example of Adductor
Head	Sternocleidomastoid	Semispinalis capitis		
Upper arm	Pectoralis major	Trapezius Latissimus dorsi	Deltoid	Pectoralis major with latissimus dorsi
Forearm	With forearm supinated: biceps brachii With forearm pronated: brachialis With semisupination or semipronation: brachioradialis	Triceps brachii		
Hand	Flexor carpi radialis and ulnaris Palmaris longus	Extensor carpi radialis, longus, and brevis Extensor carpi ulnaris	Flexor carpi radialis	Flexor carpi ulnaris
Thigh	Iliopsoas Rectus femoris (of quadriceps femoris group)	Gluteus maximus	Gluteus medius and gluteus minimus	Adductor group
Leg	Hamstrings	Quadriceps femoris group		
Foot	Tibialis anterior	Gastrocnemius Soleus	Evertors Peroneus longus Peroneus brevis	Invertor Tibialis anterior
Trunk	Iliopsoas Rectus abdominis	Sacrospinalis		

Muscles of Facial Expression and of Mastication

Muscle	Origin	Insertion	Function	Nerve Supply
MUSCLES OF FACIAL EXPRESSION				
Occipitofrontalis (epicranius)	Occipital bone	Tissues of eyebrows	Raises eyebrows, wrinkles forehead horizontally	Cranial nerve VII
Corrugator supercilii	Frontal bone (superciliary ridge)	Skin of eyebrow	Wrinkles forehead vertically	Cranial nerve VII
Orbicularis oculi	Encircles eyelid		Closes eye	Cranial nerve VII
Zygomaticus major	Zygomatic bone	Angle of mouth	Laughing (elevates angle of mouth)	Cranial nerve VII
Orbicularis oris	Encircles mouth		Draws lips together	Cranial nerve VII
Buccinator	Maxillae	Skin of sides of mouth	Permits smiling Blowing, as in playing a trumpet	Cranial nerve VII
MUSCLES OF MASTICATION				
Masseter	Zygomatic arch	Mandible (external surface)	Closes jaw	Cranial nerve V
Temporalis	Temporal bone	Mandible	Closes jaw	Cranial nerve V
Pterygoids (lateral and medial)	Undersurface of skull	Mandible (medial surface)	Grates teeth	Cranial nerve V

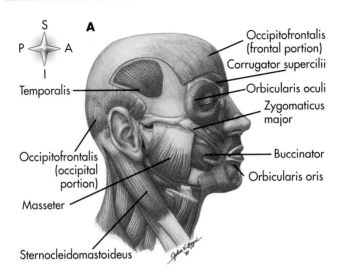

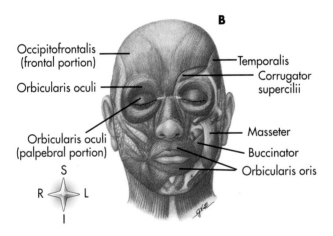

A, Lateral view of facial muscles. **B,** Anterior view of facial muscles.

Muscles That Move the Head

Muscle	Origin	Insertion	Function	Nerve Supply
Sternocleidomastoid	Sternum Clavicle	Temporal bone (mastoid process)	Flexes head (prayer muscle) One muscle alone, rotates head toward opposite side; spasm of this muscle alone or associated with trapezius called *torticollis* or *wryneck*	Accessory nerve
Semispinalis capitis	Vertebrae (transverse processes of upper six thoracic, articular processes of lower four cervical)	Occipital bone (between superior and inferior nuchal lines)	Extends head; bends it laterally	First five cervical nerves
Splenius capitis	Ligamentum nuchae	Temporal bone (mastoid process)	Extends head	Second, third, and fourth cervical nerves
Longissimus capitis	Vertebrae (spinous processes of upper three or four thoracic) Vertebrae (transverse processes of upper six thoracic, articular processes of lower four cervical)	Occipital bone Temporal bone (mastoid process)	Bends and rotates head toward same side as contracting muscle Extends head Bends and rotates head toward contracting side	Multiple innervation

ℳuscles of the Neck and Back

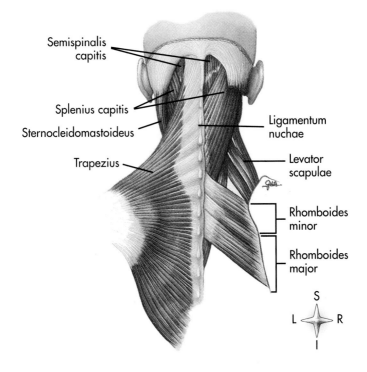

Semispinalis capitis

Splenius capitis

Sternocleidomastoideus

Trapezius

Ligamentum nuchae

Levator scapulae

Rhomboides minor

Rhomboides major

S
L — R
I

Posterior view of muscles of the neck and back.

Muscles of the Thorax

Muscle	Origin	Insertion	Function	Nerve Supply
External intercostals	Rib (lower border; forward fibers)	Rib (upper border of rib below origin)	Elevate ribs	Intercostal nerves
Internal intercostals	Rib (inner surface, lower border; backward fibers)	Rib (upper border of rib below origin)	Depress ribs	Intercostal nerves
Diaphragm	Lower circumference of thorax (of rib cage)	Central tendon of diaphragm	Enlarges thorax, causing inspiration	Phrenic nerves

Muscles of the Abdominal Wall

Muscle	Origin	Insertion	Function	Nerve Supply
External oblique	Ribs (lower eight)	Ossa coxae (iliac crest and pubis by way of inguinal ligament) Linea alba by way of an aponeurosis	Compresses abdomen Rotates trunk laterally Important postural function of all abdominal muscles is to pull front of pelvis upward, thereby flattening lumbar curve of spine; when these muscles lose their tone, common figure faults of protruding abdomen and lordosis develop	Lower seven intercostal nerves and iliohypo-gastric nerves
Internal oblique	Ossa coxae (iliac crest and inguinal ligament) Lumbodorsal fascia	Ribs (lower three) Linea alba	Same as external oblique	Last three intercostal nerves; iliohypogas-tric and ilioinguinal nerves

Continued

Muscles of the Abdominal Wall—cont'd

Muscle	Origin	Insertion	Function	Nerve Supply
Transversus abdominis	Ribs (lower six) Ossa coxae (iliac crest, inguinal ligament) Lumbodorsal fascia	Pubic bone Linea alba	Same as external oblique	Last five intercostal nerves; iliohypogastric and ilioinguinal nerves
Rectus abdominis	Ossa coxae (pubic bone and symphysis pubis)	Ribs (costal cartilage of fifth, sixth, and seventh ribs) Sternum (xiphoid process)	Same as external oblique; because abdominal muscles compress abdominal cavity, they aid in straining, defecation, forced expiration, childbirth, etc.; abdominal muscles are antagonists of diaphragm, relaxing as it contracts and vice versa Flexes trunk	Last six intercostal nerves

*M*uscles of the Trunk and Abdominal Wall

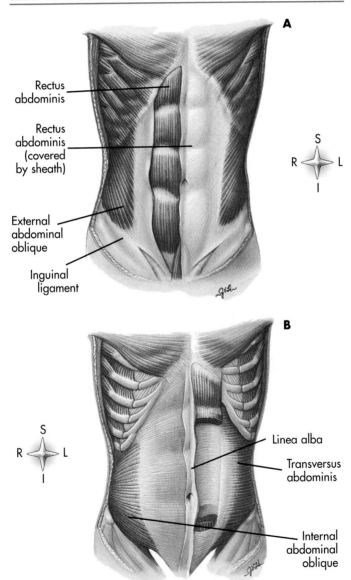

A, Anterior view of the trunk showing superficial muscles.
B, Anterior view of the trunk showing deeper muscles.

Muscles of the Pelvic Floor

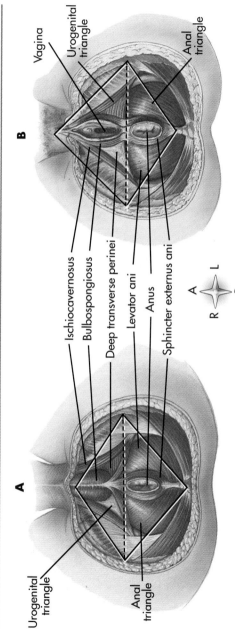

A, Male, inferior view of the pelvic floor. **B**, Female, inferior view of the pelvic floor.

Muscle	Origin	Insertion	Function	Nerve Supply
LEVATOR ANI	Pubis and spine of ischium	Coccyx	Together with coccygeus muscles form floor of pelvic cavity and support pelvic organs	Pudendal nerve
Ischiocavernosus	Ischium	Penis or clitoris	Compress base of penis or clitoris	Perineal nerve
Bulbospongiosus				
Male	Bulb of penis	Perineum and bulb of penis	Constricts urethra and erects penis	Pudendal nerve
Female	Perineum	Base of clitoris	Erects clitoris	Pudendal nerve
Deep transverse perinei	Ischium	Central tendon (median raphe)	Support pelvic floor	Pudendal nerve
Sphincter urethrae	Pubic ramus	Central tendon (median raphe)	Constrict urethra	Pudendal nerve
Sphincter externus ani	Coccyx	Central tendon (median raphe)	Close anal canal	Pudendal and S4

Muscles Acting on the Shoulder Girdle

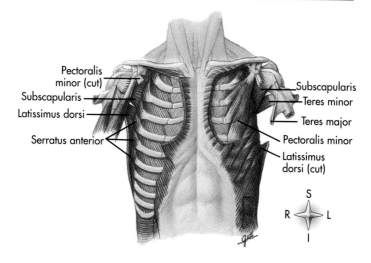

Anterior view of the shoulders—the pectoralis major has been removed on both sides. The pectoralis minor also has been removed on the right side of the illustration. (See p. 195 for a posterior view of the shoulder muscles.)

Muscle	Origin	Insertion	Function	Nerve Supply
Trapezius	Occipital bone (protuberance)	Clavicle	Raises or lowers shoulders and shrugs them	Spinal accessory; second, third, and fourth cervical nerves
	Vertebrae (cervical and thoracic)	Scapula (spine and acromion)	Extends head when occiput acts as insertion	
Pectoralis minor	Ribs (second to fifth)	Scapula (coracoid)	Pulls shoulder down and forward	Medial and lateral anterior thoracic nerves
Serratus anterior	Ribs (upper eight or nine)	Scapula (anterior surface, vertebral border)	Pulls shoulder down and forward; abducts and rotates it upward	Long thoracic nerve
Levator scapulae	C1-C4 (transverse processes)	Scapula (superior angle)	Elevates and retracts scapula and abducts neck	Dorsal scapular nerve
Rhomboideus				
Major	T1-T4	Scapula (medial border)	Retracts, rotates, fixes scapula	Dorsal scapular nerve
Minor	C6-C7	Scapula (medial border)	Retracts, rotates, elevates, and fixes scapula	Dorsal scapular nerve

$\mathcal{R}$otator Cuff Muscles

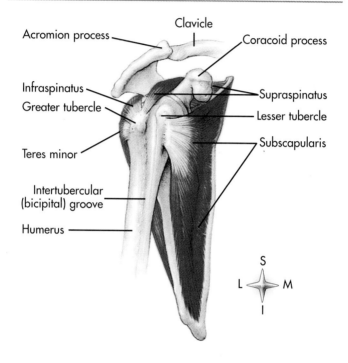

Tendons of the teres minor, infraspinatus, supraspinatus, and subscapularis muscles surround the head of the humerus.

$\mathcal{M}$uscles That Move the Upper Arm

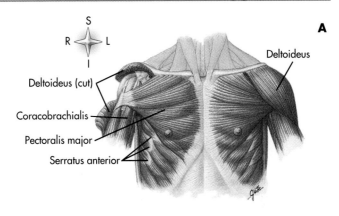

S
R ✦ L
I

A

Deltoideus

Deltoideus (cut)

Coracobrachialis

Pectoralis major

Serratus anterior

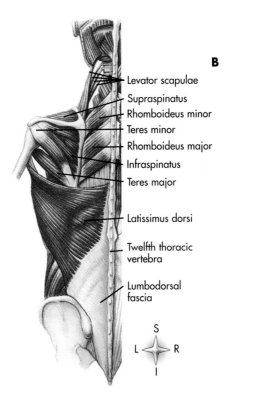

B

Levator scapulae

Supraspinatus

Rhomboideus minor

Teres minor

Rhomboideus major

Infraspinatus

Teres major

Latissimus dorsi

Twelfth thoracic vertebra

Lumbodorsal fascia

S
L ✦ R
I

A, Anterior view of the muscles that move the upper arm.
B, Posterior view of the muscles that move the upper arm.

Muscles That Move the Upper Arm—cont'd

Muscle	Origin	Insertion	Function	Nerve Supply
AXIAL*				
Pectoralis major	Clavicle (medial half) Sternum Costal cartilages of true ribs	Humerus (greater tubercle)	Flexes upper arm Adducts upper arm anteriorly; draws it across chest	Medial and lateral anterior thoracic nerves
Latissimus dorsi	Vertebrae (spines of lower thoracic, lumbar, and sacral) Ilium (crest) Lumbodorsal fascia	Humerus (intertubercular groove)	Extends upper arm Adducts upper arm posteriorly	Thoracodorsal nerve
SCAPULAR*				
Deltoid	Clavicle Scapula (spine and acromion)	Humerus (lateral side about half-way down—deltoid tubercle)	Abducts upper arm Assists in flexion and extension of upper arm	Axillary nerve

Coracobrachialis	Scapula (coracoid process)	Humerus (middle third, medial surface)	Adduction; assists in flexion and medial rotation of arm	Musculocutaneous nerve
Supraspinatus†	Scapula (supraspinous fossa)	Humerus (greater tubercle)	Assists in abducting arm	Suprascapular nerve
Teres minor†	Scapula (axillary border)	Humerus (greater tubercle)	Rotates arm outward	Axillary nerve
Teres major	Scapula (lower part, axillary border)	Humerus (upper part, anterior surface)	Assists in extension, adduction, and medial rotation of arm	Lower subscapular nerve
Infraspinatus†	Scapula (infraspinatus border)	Humerus (greater tubercle)	Rotates arm outward	Suprascapular nerve
Subscapularis†	Scapula (subscapular fossa)	Humerus (lesser tubercle)	Medial rotation	Suprascapular nerve

*Axial muscles originate on the axial skeleton.
Scapular muscles originate on the scapula.
†Muscles of the rotator cuff.

$\mathscr{M}$uscles that Move the Forearm

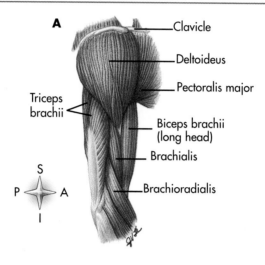

A

Clavicle

Deltoideus

Pectoralis major

Triceps brachii

Biceps brachii (long head)

Brachialis

Brachioradialis

S
P ◆ A
I

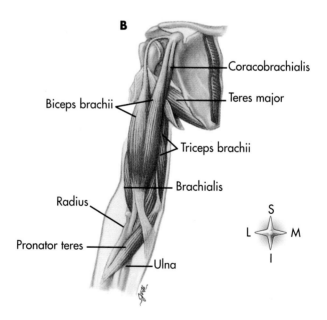

B

Coracobrachialis

Teres major

Biceps brachii

Triceps brachii

Brachialis

Radius

Pronator teres

Ulna

S
L ◆ M
I

A, Lateral view of the right shoulder and arm. **B,** Anterior view of the right shoulder and arm (deep). Deltoid and pectoralis major muscles have been removed to reveal deeper structures.

Muscles that Move the Forearm—cont'd

Muscle	Origin	Insertion	Function	Nerve Supply
FLEXORS				
Biceps brachii	Scapula (supraglenoid tuberosity)	Radius (tubercle at proximal end)	Flexes supinated forearm	Musculocutaneous nerve
	Scapula (coracoid)		Supinates forearm and hand	
Brachialis	Humerus (distal half, anterior surface)	Ulna (front of coronoid process)	Flexes pronated forearm	Musculocutaneous nerve
Brachioradialis	Humerus (above lateral epicondyle)	Radius (styloid process)	Flexes semipronated or semisupinated forearm; supinates forearm and hand	Radial nerve
EXTENSOR				
Triceps brachii	Scapula (infraglenoid tuberosity)	Ulna (olecranon process)	Extends lower arm	Radial nerve
	Humerus (posterior surface—lateral head above radial groove; medial head, below)			

Continued

*M*uscles that Move the Forearm—cont'd

Muscle	Origin	Insertion	Function	Nerve Supply
PRONATORS				
Pronator teres	Humerus (medial epicondyle) Ulna (coronoid process)	Radius (middle third of lateral surface)	Pronates and flexes forearm	Median nerve
Pronator quadratus	Ulna (distal fourth, anterior surface)	Radius (distal fourth, anterior surface)	Pronates forearm	Median nerve
SUPINATOR				
Supinator	Humerus (lateral epicondyle) Ulna (proximal fifth)	Radius (proximal third)	Supinates forearm	Radial nerve

*M*uscles That Move the Wrist, Hand, and Fingers

Muscle	Origin	Insertion	Function	Nerve Supply
EXTRINSIC				
Flexor carpi radialis	Humerus (medial epicondyle)	Second metacarpal (base of)	Flexes hand	Median nerve
			Flexes forearm	
Palmaris longus	Humerus (medial epicondyle)	Fascia of palm	Flexes hand	Median nerve
Flexor carpi ulnaris	Humerus (medial epicondyle)	Pisiform bone	Flexes hand	Ulnar nerve
	Ulna (proximal two thirds)	Third, fourth, and fifth metacarpals	Adducts hand	
Extensor carpi radialis longus	Humerus (ridge above lateral epicondyle)	Second metacarpal (base of)	Extends hand	Radial nerve
			Abducts hand (moves toward thumb side when hand supinated)	
Extensor carpi radialis brevis	Humerus (lateral epicondyle)	Second, third metacarpals (bases of)	Extends hand	Radial nerve
Extensor carpi ulnaris	Humerus (lateral epicondyle)	Fifth metacarpal (base of)	Extends hand	Radial nerve
	Ulna (proximal three fourths)		Adducts hand (moves toward little finger side when hand supinated)	

Continued

Muscles That Move the Wrist, Hand, and Fingers—cont'd

Muscle	Origin	Insertion	Function	Nerve Supply
Flexor digitorum profundus	Ulna (anterior surface)	Distal phalanges (fingers 2 to 5)	Flexes distal interphalangeal joints	Median and ulnar nerves
Flexor digitorum superficialis	Humerus (medial epicondyle) Radius Ulna (coronoid process)	Tendons of fingers	Flexes fingers	Median nerve
Extensor digitorum	Humerus (lateral epicondyle)	Phalanges (fingers 2 to 5)	Extends fingers	Radial nerve
INTRINSIC				
Opponens pollicis	Trapezium	Thumb metacarpal	Opposes thumb to fingers	Median nerve
Abductor pollicis brevis	Trapezium	Proximal phalanx of thumb	Abducts thumb	Median nerve
Adductor pollicis	Second and third metacarpals Trapezoid Capitate	Proximal phalanx of thumb	Adducts thumb	Ulnar nerve

Flexor pollicis brevis	Flexor retinaculum	Proximal phalanx of thumb	Flexes thumb	Median and ulnar nerves
Abductor digiti minimi	Pisiform	Proximal phalanx of fifth finger (base of)	Abducts fifth finger	Ulnar nerve
Flexor digiti minimi brevis	Hamate	Proximal and middle phalanx of fifth finger	Flexes fifth finger	Ulnar nerve
Opponens digiti minimi	Hamate Flexor retinaculum	Fifth metacarpal	Opposes fifth finger slightly	Ulnar nerve
Interosseous (palmar and dorsal)	Metacarpals	Proximal phalanges	Adducts second, fourth, fifth fingers (palmar) Abducts second, third, fourth fingers (dorsal)	Ulnar nerve
Lumbricales	Tendons of flexor digitorum profundus	Phalanges (2 to 5)	Flexes proximal phalanges (2 to 5) Extends middle and distal phalanges (2 to 5)	Median nerve (phalanges 2 and 3) Ulnar nerve (phalanges 4 and 5)

*M*uscles of the Forearm

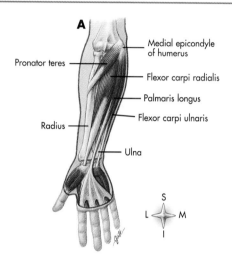

A

- Medial epicondyle of humerus
- Pronator teres
- Flexor carpi radialis
- Palmaris longus
- Flexor carpi ulnaris
- Radius
- Ulna

S
L ← → M
I

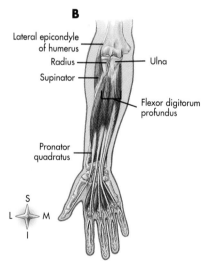

B

- Lateral epicondyle of humerus
- Radius
- Ulna
- Supinator
- Flexor digitorum profundus
- Pronator quadratus

S
L ← → M
I

A, Anterior view of the superficial muscles of the right forearm. The brachioradialis muscle has been removed. **B,** Anterior view of the right forearm showing muscles that lie deeper than those shown in **A.** Pronator teres, flexor carpi radialis and ulnaris, and palmaris longus muscles have been removed.

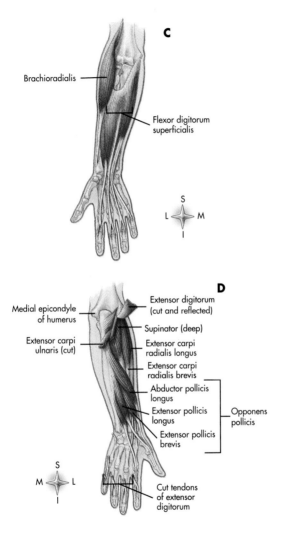

C, Anterior view of the right forearm showing muscles that lie deeper still than those in **A** and **B** on p. 214. Brachioradialis, pronator teres, flexor carpi radialis and ulnaris, palmaris longus, and flexor digitorum superficialis muscles have been removed. **D,** Posterior view of the right forearm showing deep muscles of the right forearm. Extensor digitorum, extensor digiti minimi, and extensor carpi ulnaris muscles have been cut to reveal deeper muscles.

Intrinsic Muscles of the Hand

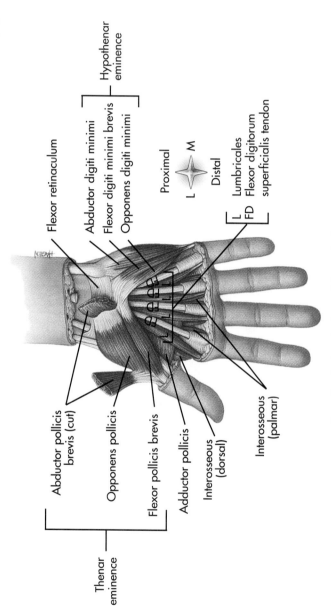

Flexor retinaculum

Abductor digiti minimi
Flexor digiti minimi brevis
Opponens digiti minimi

Hypothenar eminence

Proximal

L — M

Distal

Lumbricales
Flexor digitorum
superficialis tendon

L
FD

Abductor pollicis
brevis (cut)

Opponens pollicis

Flexor pollicis brevis

Adductor pollicis

Interosseous
(dorsal)

Interosseous
(palmar)

Thenar
eminence

Anterior (palmar) view of the right hand.

*C*arpal Tunnel

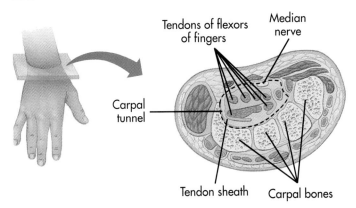

The median nerve and muscles that flex the fingers pass through a concavity in the wrist called the *carpal tunnel*.

Muscles That Move the Thigh

Muscle	Origin	Insertion	Function	Nerve Supply
ILIOPSOAS (ILIACUS, PSOAS MAJOR, AND PSOAS MINOR)	Ilium (iliac fossa) Vertebrae (bodies of twelfth thoracic to fifth lumbar)	Femur (lesser trochanter)	Flexes thigh Flexes trunk (when femur acts as origin)	Femoral and second to fourth lumbar nerves
RECTUS FEMORIS	Ilium (anterior, inferior spine)	Tibia (by way of patellar tendon)	Flexes thigh Extends lower leg	Femoral nerve
GLUTEAL GROUP				
Maximum	Ilium (crest and posterior surface) Sacrum and coccyx (posterior surface) Sacrotuberous ligament	Femur (gluteal tuberosity) Iliotibial tract	Extends thigh—rotates outward	Inferior gluteal nerve
Medius	Ilium (lateral surface)	Femur (greater trochanter)	Abducts thigh—rotates outward; stabilizes pelvis on femur	Superior gluteal nerve

Muscle	Origin	Insertion	Function	Nerve
GLUTEAL GROUP—CONT'D				
Minimus	Ilium (lateral surface)	Femur (greater trochanter)	Abducts thigh; stabilizes pelvis on femur. Rotates thigh medially	Superior gluteal nerve
TENSOR FASCIAE LATAE	Ilium (anterior part of crest)	Tibia (by way of iliotibial tract)	Abducts thigh. Tightens iliotibial tract	Superior gluteal nerve
ADDUCTOR GROUP				
Brevis	Pubic bone	Femur (linea aspera)	Adducts thigh	Obturator nerve
Longus	Pubic bone	Femur (linea aspera)	Adducts thigh	Obturator nerve
Magnus	Pubic bone	Femur (linea aspera)	Adducts thigh	Obturator nerve
GRACILIS	Pubic bone (just below symphysis)	Tibia (medial surface behind sartorius)	Adducts thigh and flexes and adducts leg	Obturator nerve

Iliopsoas Muscle

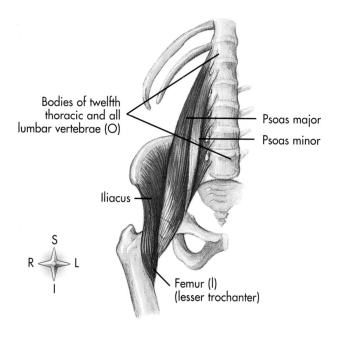

Bodies of twelfth thoracic and all lumbar vertebrae (O)

Psoas major

Psoas minor

Iliacus

S
R ✛ L
I

Femur (I) (lesser trochanter)

The iliopsoas muscle complex includes the iliacus, psoas major, and psoas minor muscles. *O* indicates the point of origin of the muscle. *I* indicates the insertion point of the muscle.

*M*uscles of the Anterior Thigh

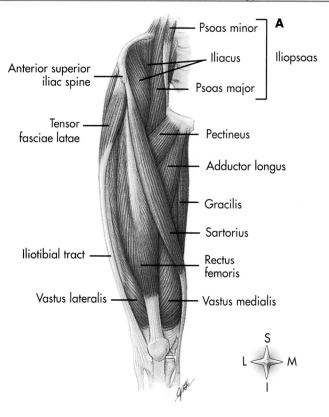

Psoas minor
Iliacus | Iliopsoas
Psoas major

A

Anterior superior
iliac spine

Tensor
fasciae latae

Pectineus

Adductor longus

Gracilis

Sartorius

Iliotibial tract

Rectus
femoris

Vastus lateralis

Vastus medialis

S
L ⟷ M
I

A, Anterior view of the right thigh.
Continued

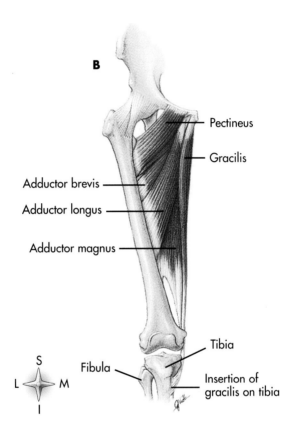

B, Adductor region of the right thigh. Tensor fasciae latae, sartorius, and quadriceps muscles have been removed.

Muscles That Adduct the Thigh

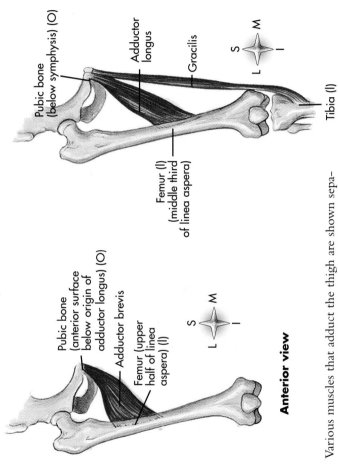

Pubic bone (below symphysis) (O)

Adductor longus

Gracilis

Femur (I) (middle third of linea aspera)

Tibia (I)

Anterior view

Pubic bone (anterior surface below origin of adductor longus) (O)

Adductor brevis

Femur (upper half of linea aspera) (I)

Anterior view

Various muscles that adduct the thigh are shown separately for the sake of clarity.

Continued

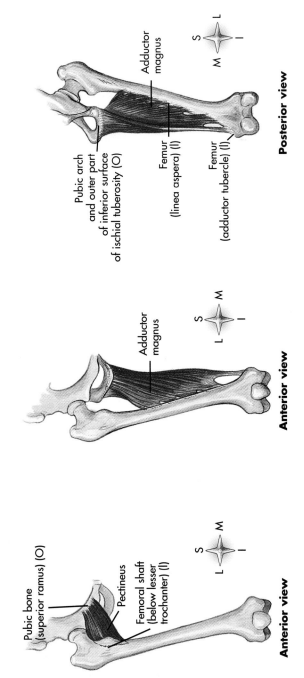

Various muscles that adduct the thigh are shown separately for the sake of clarity.

*M*uscles That Move the Lower Leg

Muscle	Origin	Insertion	Function	Nerve Supply
QUADRICEPS FEMORIS GROUP				
Rectus femoris	Ilium (anterior inferior spine)	Tibia (by way of patellar tendon)	Flexes thigh; Extends leg	Femoral nerve
Vastus lateralis	Femur (linea aspera)	Tibia (by way of patellar tendon)	Extends leg	Femoral nerve
Vastus medialis	Femur	Tibia (by way of patellar tendon)	Extends leg	Femoral nerve
Vastus intermedius	Femur (anterior surface)	Tibia (by way of patellar tendon)	Extends leg	Femoral nerve
SARTORIUS	Coxal (anterior, superior iliac spines)	Tibia (medial surface of upper end of shaft)	Adducts and flexes leg; Permits crossing of legs tailor fashion	Femoral nerve
HAMSTRING GROUP				
Biceps femoris	Ischium (tuberosity)	Fibula (head of)	Flexes leg	Hamstring nerve (branch of sciatic nerve)
	Femur (linea aspera)	Tibia (lateral condyle)	Extends thigh	Hamstring nerve
Semitendinosus	Ischium (tuberosity)	Tibia (proximal end, medial surface)	Extends thigh	Hamstring nerve
Semimembranosus	Ischium (tuberosity)	Tibia (medial condyle)	Extends thigh	Hamstring nerve

Gluteal Muscles

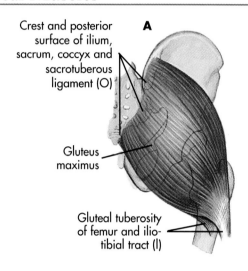

Crest and posterior surface of ilium, sacrum, coccyx and sacrotuberous ligament (O)

A

Gluteus maximus

Gluteal tuberosity of femur and ilio-tibial tract (I)

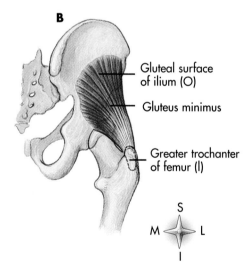

B

Gluteal surface of ilium (O)

Gluteus minimus

Greater trochanter of femur (I)

S

M — L

I

A, Gluteus maximus. **B,** Gluteus minimus.

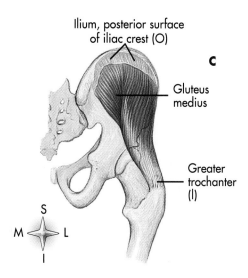

Ilium, posterior surface of iliac crest (O)

C

Gluteus medius

Greater trochanter (I)

S

M ◄✦► L

I

C, Gluteus medius.

Muscles That Move the Foot

Muscle	Origin	Insertion	Function	Nerve Supply
EXTRINSIC				
Tibialis anterior	Tibia (lateral condyle of upper body)	Tarsal (first cuneiform) Metatarsal (base of first)	Flexes foot Inverts foot	Common and deep peroneal nerves
Gastrocnemius	Femur (condyles)	Tarsal (calcaneus by way of Achilles tendon)	Extends foot Flexes lower leg	Tibial nerve (branch of sciatic nerve)
Soleus	Tibia (underneath gastrocnemius) Fibula	Tarsal (calcaneus by way of Achilles tendon)	Extends foot (plantar flexion)	Tibial nerve
Peroneus longus	Tibia (lateral condyle) Fibula (head and shaft)	First cuneiform Base of first metatarsal	Extends foot (plantar flexion) Everts foot	Common peroneal nerve
Peroneus brevis	Fibula (lower two thirds of lateral surface of shaft)	Fifth metatarsal (tubercle, dorsal surface)	Everts foot Flexes foot	Superficial peroneal nerve
Peroneus tertius	Fibula (distal third)	Fourth and fifth metatarsals (bases of)	Flexes foot Everts foot	Deep peroneal nerve
Extensor digitorum longus	Tibia (lateral condyle) Fibula (anterior surface)	Second and third phalanges (four lateral toes)	Dorsiflexion of foot; extension of toes	Deep peroneal nerve

INTRINSIC

Muscle	Origin	Insertion	Action	Nerve
Lumbricales	Tendons of flexor digitorum longus	Phalanges (2 to 5)	Flex proximal phalanges Extend middle and distal phalanges	Lateral and medial plantar nerve
Flexor digiti minimi brevis	Fifth metatarsal	Proximal phalanx of fifth toe	Flexes fifth (small) toe	Lateral plantar nerve
Flexor hallucis brevis	Cuboid Medial and lateral cuneiform	Proximal phalanx of first (great) toe	Flexes first (great) toe	Medial and lateral plantar nerve
Flexor digitorum brevis	Calcaneous Plantar fascia	Middle phalanges of toes (2 to 5)	Flexes second through fifth toes	Medial plantar nerve
Abductor digiti minimi	Calcaneous	Proximal phalanx of fifth (small) toe	Abducts fifth (small) toe Flexes fifth toe	Lateral plantar nerve
Abductor hallucis	Calcaneous	First (great) toe	Abducts first (great) toe	Medial plantar nerve

Superficial Muscles of the Leg

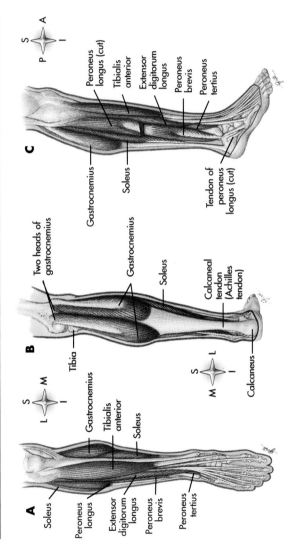

A, Anterior view of the lower right leg. **B,** Posterior view of the lower right leg. **C,** Lateral view of the lower right leg.

$\mathcal{I}$ntrinsic Muscles of the Foot

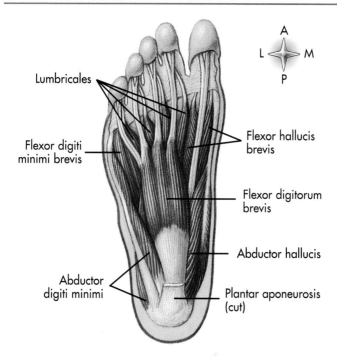

Lumbricales

Flexor digiti
minimi brevis

Flexor hallucis
brevis

Flexor digitorum
brevis

Abductor hallucis

Abductor
digiti minimi

Plantar aponeurosis
(cut)

8

Nervous
System

The nervous system is organized to detect changes (stimuli) in the internal and external environment, evaluate that information, and possibly respond by initiating changes in muscles or glands. To make this complex network of information lines and processing circuits easier to understand, biologists have subdivided the nervous system into smaller "systems" and "divisions." The nervous system can be divided in various ways: according to structure, direction of information flow, or control of effectors.

$\mathcal{O}$rganizational Plan of the Nervous System

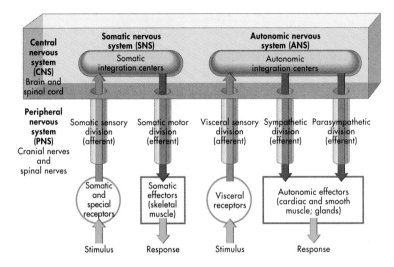

This diagram summarizes the scheme used by most neurobiologists in studying the nervous system. Both the somatic nervous system (SNS) and the autonomic nervous system (ANS) include components in the central nervous system (CNS) and peripheral nervous system (PNS). Somatic sensory pathways conduct information toward integrators in the CNS, and somatic motor pathways conduct information toward somatic effectors. In the ANS, visceral sensory pathways conduct information toward CNS integrators, whereas the sympathetic and parasympathetic pathways conduct information toward autonomic effectors.

*T*ypes of Glia

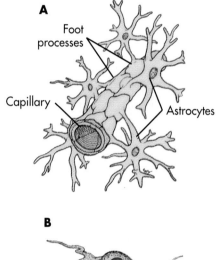

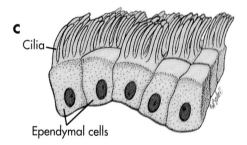

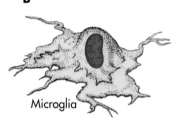

Glia (neuroglia) are the nonconducting "support cells" of nervous tissue. **A,** Astrocytes attached to the outside of a capillary blood vessel in the brain. **B,** A phagocytic microglial cell. **C,** Ciliated ependymal cells forming a sheet that usually lines fluid cavities in the brain.

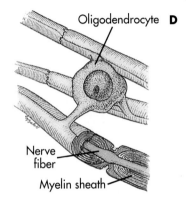

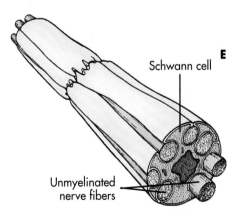

D, An oligodendrocyte with processes that wrap around nerve fibers in the CNS to form myelin sheaths. **E,** A Schwann cell supporting a bundle of nerve fibers in the PNS. *Continued*

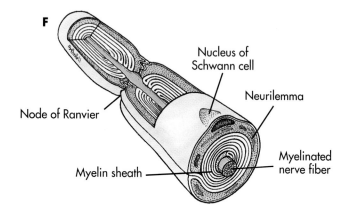

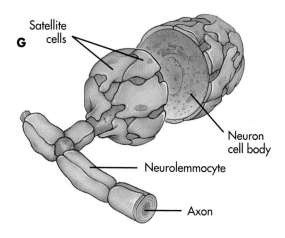

F, Another type of Schwann cell wrapping around a peripheral nerve fiber to form a thick myelin sheath. **G,** Satellite cells, another type of Schwann cell, surround and support cell bodies of neurons in the PNS.

Structure of a Typical Neuron

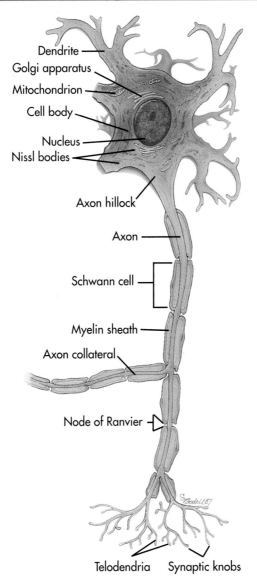

Dendrite

Golgi apparatus

Mitochondrion

Cell body

Nucleus

Nissl bodies

Axon hillock

Axon

Schwann cell

Myelin sheath

Axon collateral

Node of Ranvier

Telodendria   Synaptic knobs

Structural Classification of Neurons

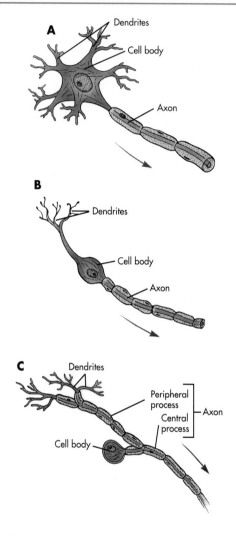

A, Multipolar neuron: neuron with multiple extensions from the cell body. **B,** Bipolar neuron: neuron with exactly two extensions from the cell body. **C,** Unipolar (pseudounipolar) neuron: neuron with only one extension from the cell body. The central process is an axon; the peripheral process is a modified axon with branched dendrites at its extremity. (The *arrows* show the direction of impulse travel.)

Functional Classification of Neurons

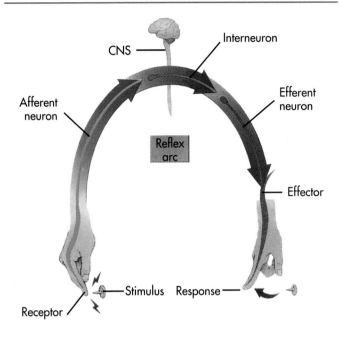

Neurons can be classified according to the direction in which they conduct impulses. Notice that the most basic route of signal conduction follows a pattern called the reflex arc.

The Nerve

Nerves are bundles of peripheral nerve fibers held together by several layers of connective tissues.

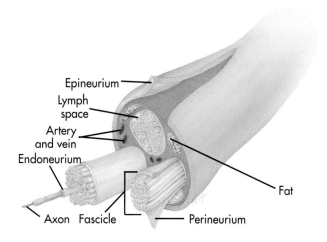

Epineurium

Lymph space

Artery and vein

Endoneurium

Axon Fascicle

Fat

Perineurium

Each nerve contains axons bundled into fascicles. A connective tissue epineurium wraps the entire nerve. Perineurium surrounds each fascicle.

*M*embrane Potential

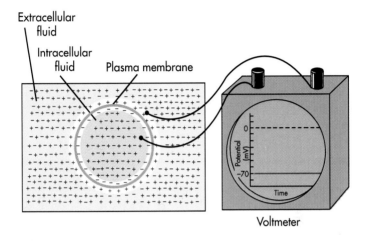

Extracellular fluid

Intracellular fluid

Plasma membrane

Voltmeter

The diagram *on the left* represents a cell maintaining a very slight difference in the concentration of oppositely charged ions across its plasma membrane. The voltmeter records the magnitude of electrical difference over time, which, in this case, does not fluctuate from -70 mV (voltage recorded over time as a *red line*).

*D*epolarization and Repolarization

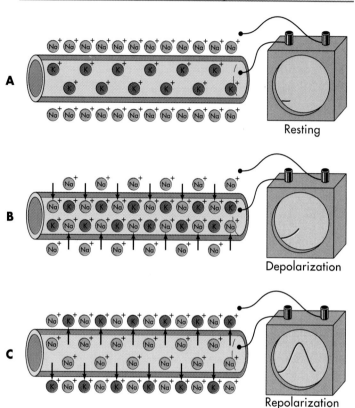

A, Resting membrane potential (RMP) results from an excess of positive ions on the outer surface of the plasma membrane. More Na^+ ions are on the outside of the membrane than K^+ ions are on the inside of the membrane. **B,** Depolarization of a membrane occurs when Na^+ channels open, allowing Na^+ to move to an area of lower concentration (and more negative charge) *inside* the cell—reversing the polarity to an inside-positive state. **C,** Repolarization of a membrane occurs when K^+ channels then open, allowing K^+ to move to an area of lower concentration (and more negative charge) *outside* the cell—reversing the polarity back to an inside-negative state. Each voltmeter records the changing membrane potential as a *red line*.

The Action Potential

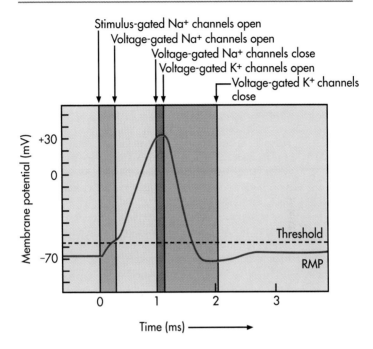

Changes in membrane potential in a local area of a neuron's membrane result from changes in membrane permeability.

*S*teps of the Mechanism that Produces an Action Potential

Step	Description
1	A stimulus triggers stimulus-gated Na^+ channels to open and allow inward Na^+ diffusion. This causes the membrane to depolarize.
2	As the threshold potential is reached, voltage-gated Na^+ channels open.
3	As more Na^+ enters the cell through voltage-gated Na^+ channels, the membrane depolarizes even further.
4	The magnitude of the action potential peaks (at +30 mV) when voltage-gated Na^+ channels close.
5	Repolarization begins when voltage-gated K^+ channels open, allowing outward diffusion of K^+.
6	After a brief period of hyperpolarization, the resting potential is restored by the sodium-potassium pump and the return of ion channels to their resting state.

*R*efractory Period

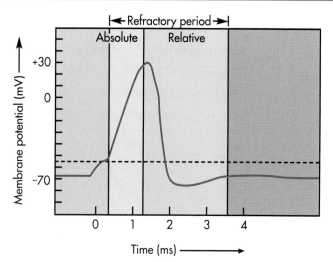

During the absolute refractory period, the membrane will not respond to any stimulus. During the relative refractory period, however, a very strong stimulus may elicit a response in the membrane.

The Chemical Synapse

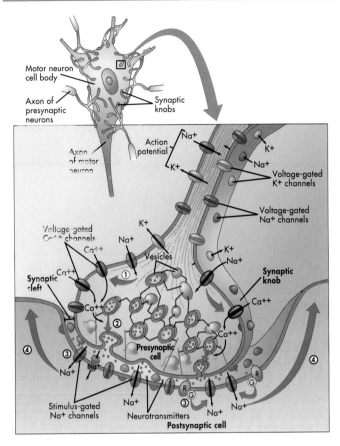

The diagram shows the detail of a synaptic knob, or axon terminal, of presynaptic neuron, the plasma membrane of a postsynaptic neuron, and a synaptic cleft. On the arrival of an action potential at a synaptic knob, voltage-gated Ca^{++} channels open and allow extracellular Ca^{++} to diffuse into the presynaptic cell (*step 1*). In *step 2*, the Ca^{++} triggers the rapid exocytosis of neurotransmitter molecules from vesicles in the knob. In *step 3*, neurotransmitter diffuses into the synaptic cleft and binds to receptor molecules in the plasma membrane of the postsynaptic neuron. The postsynaptic receptors directly or indirectly trigger the opening of stimulus-gated ion channels, initiating a local potential in the postsynaptic neuron. In *step 4*, the local potential may move toward the axon, where an action potential may begin.

*D*irect Stimulation of Postsynaptic Receptor

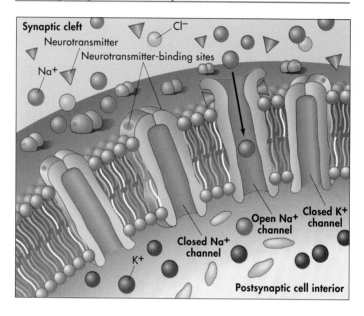

Some neurotransmitters, such as acetylcholine (ACh), initiate nerve signals by binding directly to one or both neurotransmitter-binding sites on the stimulus-gated ion channel. Such binding causes the channel to change its shape to an open position. When the neurotransmitter is removed, the channel again closes.

$\mathcal{G}$ Protein–Linked Stimulation of Postsynaptic Receptor

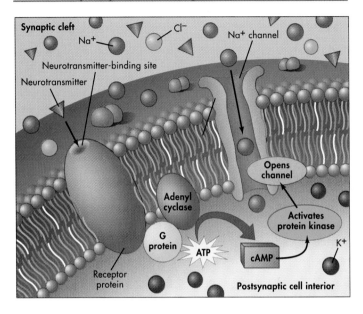

Norepinephrine and many other neurotransmitters initiate nerve signals indirectly by binding to a receptor linked to a G protein that changes shape to activate the enzyme adenylate cyclase, which in turn catalyzes the conversion of adenosine triphosphate (ATP) to cyclic adenosine monophosphate (cAMP). cAMP is a "second messenger" that induces a change in the shape of a stimulus–gated channel. Compare this with the previous illustration.

Examples of Neurotransmitters

Neurotransmitter	Location*	Function*
ACETYLCHOLINE	Junctions with motor effectors (muscles, glands); many parts of brain	Excitatory or inhibitory; involved in memory
AMINES		
Serotonin	Several regions of the central nervous system CNS	Mostly inhibitory; involved in moods and emotions, sleep
Histamine	Brain	Mostly excitatory; involved in emotions and regulation of body temperature and water balance
Dopamine	Brain; autonomic system	Mostly inhibitory; involved in emotions/moods and in regulating motor control
Epinephrine	Several areas of the CNS and in the sympathetic division of the autonomic nervous system (ANS)	Excitatory or inhibitory; acts as a hormone when secreted by sympathetic neurosecretory cells of the adrenal gland
Norepinephrine	Several areas of the CNS and in the sympathetic division of the ANS	Excitatory or inhibitory; regulates sympathetic effectors; in brain, involved in emotional responses

AMINO ACIDS		
Glutamate (glutamic acid)	CNS	Excitatory; most common excitatory neurotransmitter in CNS
Gamma–aminobutyric acid (GABA)	Brain	Inhibitory; most common inhibitory neurotransmitter in brain
Glycine	Spinal cord	Inhibitory; most common inhibitory neurotransmitter in spinal cord
NEUROPEPTIDES		
Vasoactive intestinal peptide (VIP)	Brain; some ANS and sensory fibers; retina; gastrointestinal tract	Function in nervous system uncertain
Cholecystokinin (CCK)	Brain; retina	Function in nervous system uncertain
Substance P	Brain, spinal cord, sensory pain pathways; gastrointestinal tract	Mostly excitatory; transmits pain information
Enkephalins	Several regions of CNS; retina; intestinal tract	Mostly inhibitory; act like opiates to block pain
Endorphins	Several regions of CNS; retina; intestinal tract	Mostly inhibitory; act like opiates to block pain
GASES		
Nitric oxide (NO)	Parasympathetic nervous system (PNS); parasympathetic fibers in penis, gastrointestinal tract, respiratory tract, CNS (brain)	Probably affects internal function of postsynaptic cell, with no direct influence on postsynaptic potential

*These are examples only; most of these neurotransmitters are also found in other locations, and many have additional functions.

The Central Nervous System

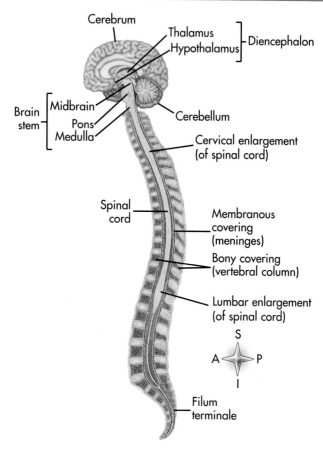

Details of both the brain and the spinal cord are shown in the above illustration.

Coverings of the Brain

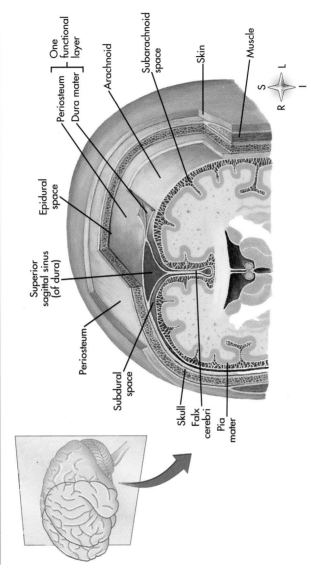

Periosteum
Dura mater
} One functional layer

Arachnoid

Subarachnoid space

Skin

Muscle

S
R — L
I

Epidural space

Superior sagittal sinus (of dura)

Periosteum

Subdural space

Skull

Falx cerebri

Pia mater

This illustration shows the frontal section of the superior portion of the head, as viewed from the front. Both the bony and the membranous coverings of the brain can be seen.

Coverings of the Spinal Cord

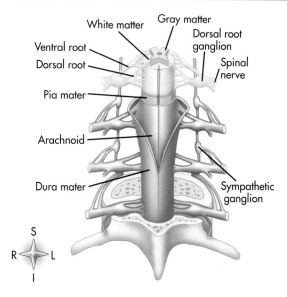

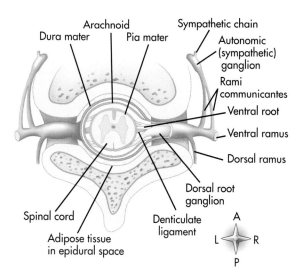

The dura mater is shown in a *natural color.* Notice how it extends to cover the spinal nerve roots and nerves. The arachnoid is highlighted in *blue* and the pia mater in *pink.*

Fluid Spaces of the Brain

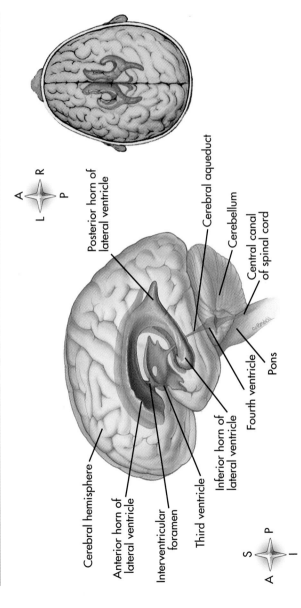

Cerebral hemisphere

Anterior horn of
lateral ventricle

Interventricular
foramen

Third ventricle

Inferior horn of
lateral ventricle

Fourth ventricle

Pons

Central canal
of spinal cord

Cerebellum

Cerebral aqueduct

Posterior horn of
lateral ventricle

The *large figure* shows the ventricles highlighted within the brain in a left lateral view. The *small figure* shows the ventricles from above.

Flow of Cerebrospinal Fluid

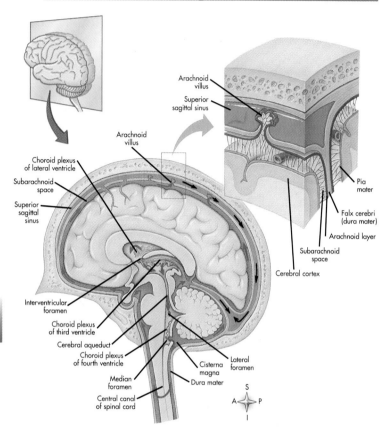

The fluid produced by filtration of blood by the choroid plexus of each ventricle flows inferiorly through the lateral ventricles, interventricular foramen, third ventricle, cerebral aqueduct, fourth ventricle, and subarachnoid space and to the blood.

Spinal Cord

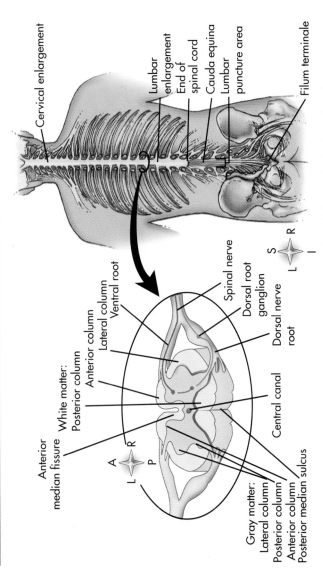

Cervical enlargement

Lumbar enlargement
End of spinal cord
Cauda equina
Lumbar puncture area
Filium terminale

Anterior median fissure
White matter:
Posterior column
Anterior column
Lateral column
Ventral root

Spinal nerve
Dorsal root ganglion
Dorsal nerve root

Central canal

Gray matter:
Lateral column
Posterior column
Anterior column
Posterior median sulcus

The *inset* illustrates a transverse section of the spinal cord shown in the broader view.

*M*ajor Tracts of the Spinal Cord

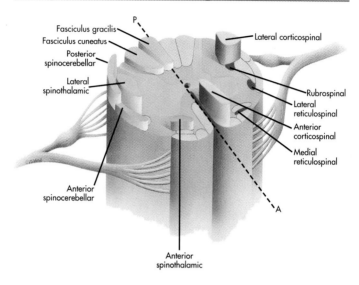

Fasciculus gracilis
Fasciculus cuneatus
Posterior spinocerebellar
Lateral spinothalamic
Anterior spinocerebellar
P
Lateral corticospinal
Rubrospinal
Lateral reticulospinal
Anterior corticospinal
Medial reticulospinal
A
Anterior spinothalamic

The major ascending (sensory) tracts, shown only *on the left* here, are highlighted in *blue*. The major descending (motor) tracts, shown only *on the right*, are highlighted in *red*. The *broken line* indicates the anterior/posterior orientation angle.

Major Ascending Tracts of the Spinal Cord

Name	Function	Location	Origin*	Termination†
LATERAL SPINOTHALAMIC	Pain, temperature, and crude touch opposite side	Lateral white columns	Posterior gray column opposite side	Thalamus
ANTERIOR SPINOTHALAMIC	Crude touch and pressure	Anterior white columns	Posterior gray column opposite side	Thalamus
FASCICULI GRACILIS AND CUNEATUS	Discriminating touch and pressure sensations, including vibration, stereognosis, and two-point discrimination; also conscious kinesthesia	Posterior white columns	Spinal ganglia same side	Medulla
ANTERIOR AND POSTERIOR SPINOCEREBELLAR	Unconscious kinesthesia	Lateral white columns	Anterior or posterior gray column	Cerebellum

*Location of cell bodies of neurons from which axons of tract arise.
†Structure in which axons of tract terminate.

*M*ajor Descending Tracts of the Spinal Cord

Name	Function	Location	Origin*	Termination†
LATERAL CORTICOSPINAL (OR CROSSED PYRAMIDAL)	Voluntary movement, contraction of individual or small groups of muscles, particularly those moving hands, fingers, feet, and toes of opposite side	Lateral white columns	Motor areas or cerebral cortex opposite side from tract location in cord	Lateral or anterior gray columns
ANTERIOR CORTICOSPINAL (DIRECT PYRAMIDAL)	Same as lateral corticospinal except mainly muscles of same side	Anterior white columns	Motor cortex but on same side as location in cord	Lateral or anterior gray columns
LATERAL RETICULOSPINAL	Mainly facilitatory influence on motor neurons to skeletal muscles	Lateral white columns	Reticular formation, midbrain, pons, and medulla	Lateral or anterior gray columns
MEDIAL RETICULOSPINAL	Mainly inhibitory influence on motor neurons to skeletal muscles	Anterior white columns	Reticular formation, medulla mainly	Lateral or anterior gray columns
RUBROSPINAL	Coordination of body movement and posture	Lateral white columns	Red nucleus (of midbrain)	Lateral or anterior gray columns

*Location of cell bodies of neurons from which axons of tract arise.
†Structure in which axons of tract terminate.

Divisions of the Brain

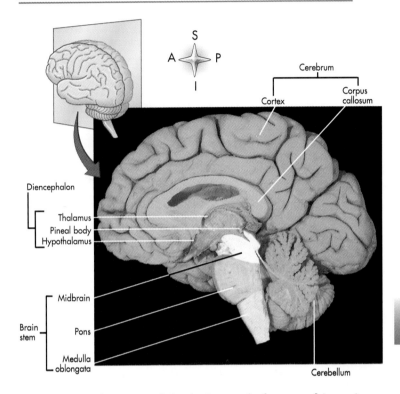

A midsagittal section of the brain reveals features of its major divisions.

Human Brain Specimens

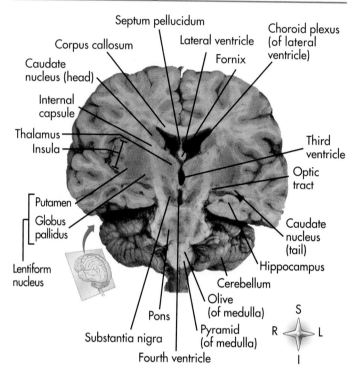

Oblique frontal section of the human brain.

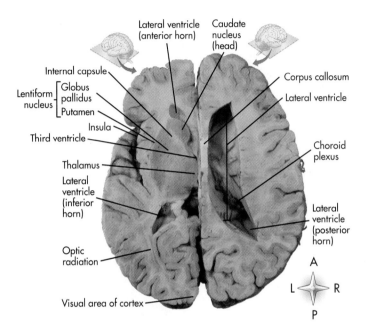

Horizontal sections of the human brain. The left section is slightly inferior to the right section.

The Brainstem and Diencephalon

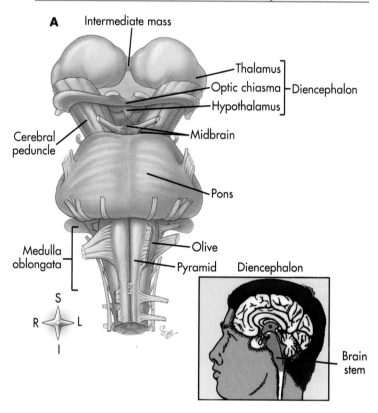

A, Anterior aspect of the brainstem and diencephalon.

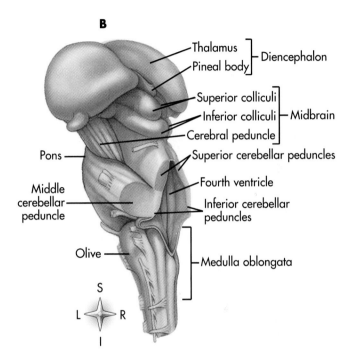

B, Posterior aspect (shifted slightly to the lateral).

*𝒯*he Cerebellum

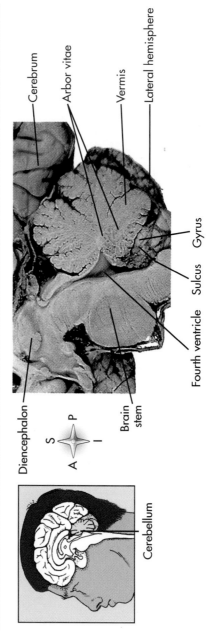

This midsagittal section shows features of the cerebellum and surrounding structures of the brain.

*C*oordinating Function
of the Cerebellum

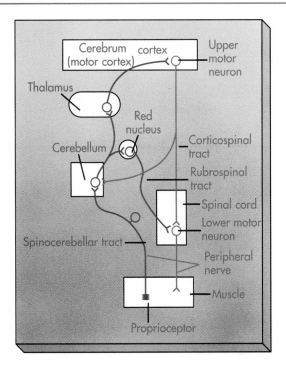

Impulses from the motor control areas of the cerebrum travel down to skeletal muscle tissue and to the cerebellum at the same time. The cerebellum, which also receives sensory information from the muscle tissue, compares the intended movement to the actual movement. It then sends impulses to both the cerebrum and the muscle tissue, thus coordinating and "smoothing" muscle activity.

Diencephalon and Surrounding Structures

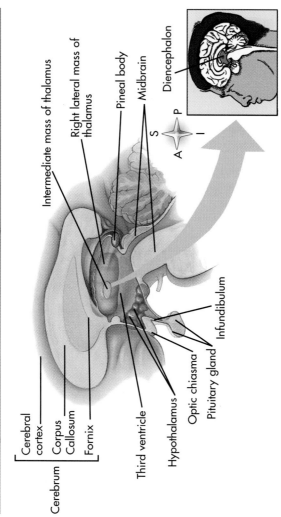

Cerebrum
- Cerebral cortex
- Corpus Callosum
- Fornix

Intermediate mass of thalamus

Right lateral mass of thalamus

Pineal body

Midbrain

Diencephalon

Third ventricle

Hypothalamus

Optic chiasma

Pituitary gland

Infundibulum

This midsagittal section highlights the largest regions of the diencephalon, the thalamus and hypothalamus, but also shows the smaller optic chiasma and pineal body. Note the position of the diencephalon between the midbrain and the cerebrum. Compare this view of the diencephalon with that on p. 262.

Left Hemisphere of the Cerebrum

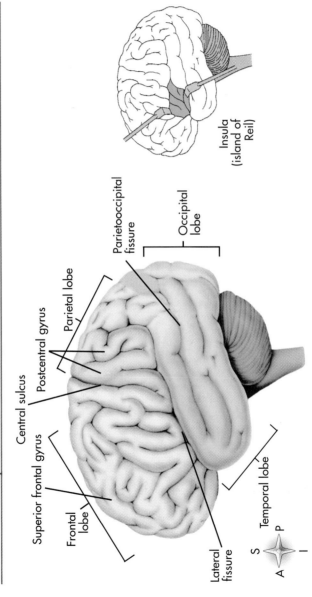

Central sulcus

Postcentral gyrus

Parietal lobe

Parietooccipital fissure

Occipital lobe

Superior frontal gyrus

Frontal lobe

Lateral fissure

Temporal lobe

Insula (island of Reil)

S
A — P
I

This illustration shows the lateral surface of the left hemisphere of the cerebrum. Each lobe of the cerebrum is *highlighted in color.*

*C*erebral Nuclei

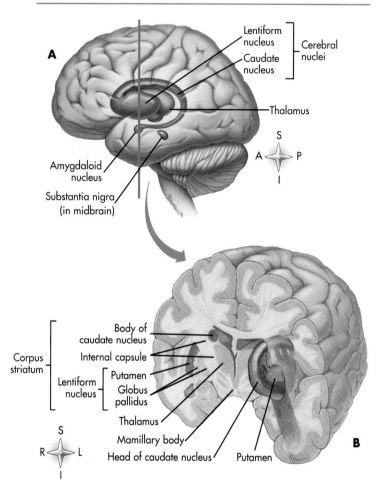

A, The cerebral nuclei seen through the cortex of the left cerebral hemisphere. **B,** The cerebral nuclei seen in a frontal (coronal) section of the brain.

*F*unctional Areas of the Cerebral Cortex

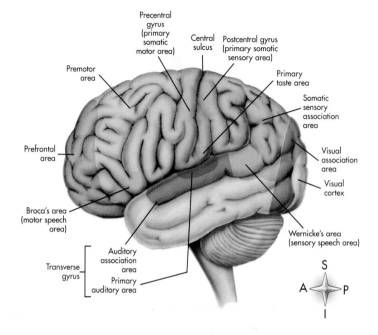

Precentral gyrus (primary somatic motor area)

Central sulcus

Postcentral gyrus (primary somatic sensory area)

Premotor area

Primary taste area

Somatic sensory association area

Prefrontal area

Visual association area

Visual cortex

Broca's area (motor speech area)

Wernicke's area (sensory speech area)

Transverse gyrus

Auditory association area

Primary auditory area

S
A P
I

Primary Somatic Sensory and Motor Areas of the Cortex

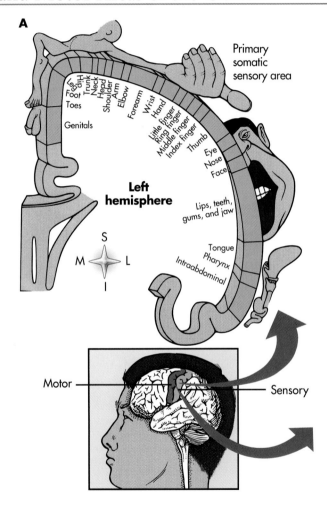

A, Primary somatic sensory areas of the cortex.

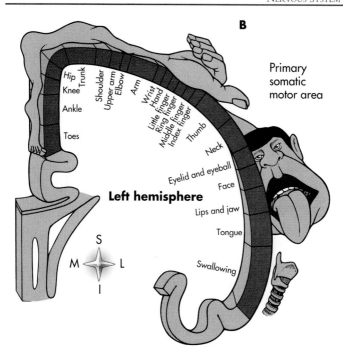

B

Primary
somatic
motor area

Left hemisphere

B, Motor areas of the cortex. The body parts illustrated here show which parts of the body are "mapped" to specific areas of each cortical area. The exaggerated face indicates that more cortical area is devoted to processing information to/from the many receptors and motor units of the face than for the leg or arm, for example.

Structures of the Limbic System

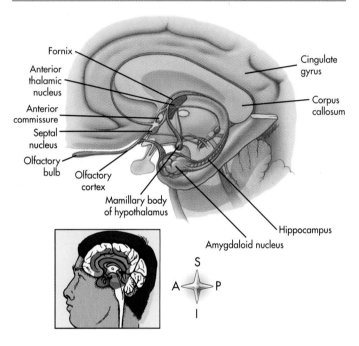

Fornix

Anterior thalamic nucleus

Anterior commissure

Septal nucleus

Olfactory bulb

Olfactory cortex

Mamillary body of hypothalamus

Cingulate gyrus

Corpus callosum

Hippocampus

Amygdaloid nucleus

S
A — P
I

The Electroencephalogram

Diagnosis and evaluation of epilepsy or any seizure disorder often rely on electroencephalography (EEG).

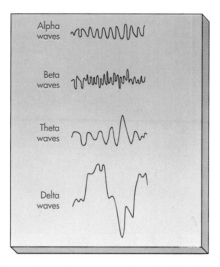

The illustration above shows examples of alpha, beta, theta, and delta waves seen on an EEG.

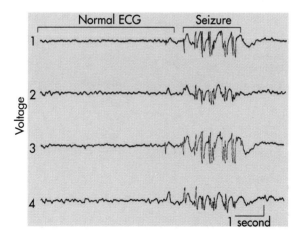

A normal EEG shows the moderate rise and fall of voltage in various parts of the brain, but a seizure manifests as an explosive increase in the size and frequency of voltage fluctuations. Different classifications of seizure disorders are based on the location(s) and the duration of these changes in brain activity.

Examples of Somatic Sensory Pathways

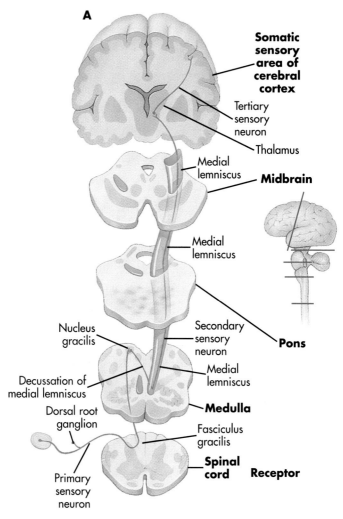

A, A pathway of the medial lemniscal system that conducts information about discriminating touch and kinesthesia.

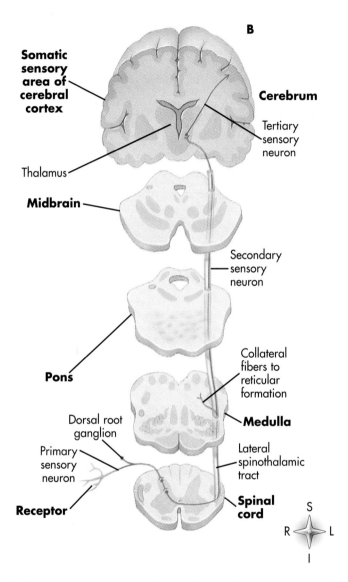

B, A spinothalmic pathway that conducts information about pain and temperature.

*E*xamples of Somatic Motor Pathways

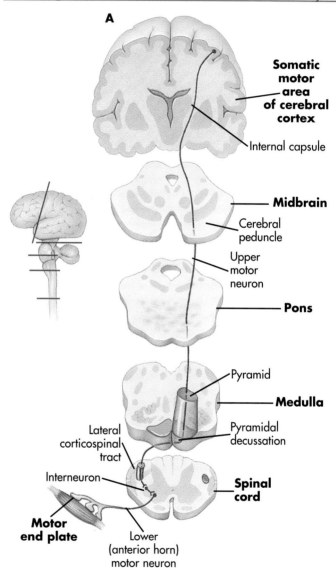

A

Somatic
motor
area
of cerebral
cortex

Internal capsule

Midbrain

Cerebral
peduncle

Upper
motor
neuron

Pons

Pyramid

Medulla

Lateral
corticospinal
tract

Pyramidal
decussation

Interneuron

**Spinal
cord**

**Motor
end plate**

Lower
(anterior horn)
motor neuron

A, A pyramidal pathway, through the lateral corticospinal tract.

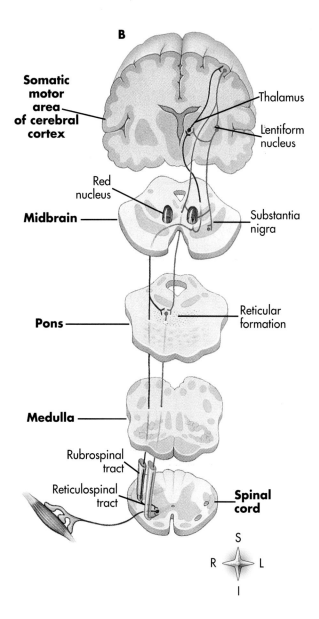

B, Extrapyramidal pathways, through the rubrospinal and reticulospinal tracts.

Spinal Nerves

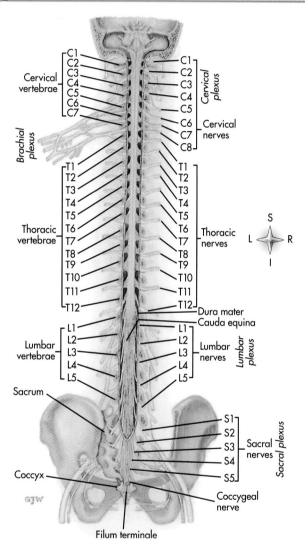

Cervical vertebrae — C1, C2, C3, C4, C5, C6, C7

Brachial plexus

Thoracic vertebrae — T1, T2, T3, T4, T5, T6, T7, T8, T9, T10, T11, T12

Lumbar vertebrae — L1, L2, L3, L4, L5

Sacrum

Coccyx

Filum terminale

Cervical plexus — C1, C2, C3, C4, C5

Cervical nerves — C6, C7, C8

Thoracic nerves — T1, T2, T3, T4, T5, T6, T7, T8, T9, T10, T11, T12

Dura mater

Cauda equina

Lumbar plexus / Lumbar nerves — L1, L2, L3, L4, L5

Sacral nerves / Sacral plexus — S1, S2, S3, S4, S5

Coccygeal nerve

S
L — R
I

GJW

Each of 31 pairs of spinal nerves exits the spinal cavity from the intervertebral foramina. The names of the vertebrae are given *on the left* and the names of the corresponding spinal nerves *on the right*. Notice that after leaving the spinal cavity, many of the spinal nerves interconnect to form networks called plexuses.

*R*ami of the Spinal Nerves

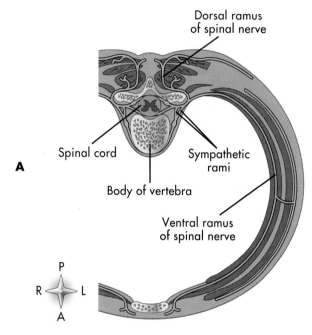

Dorsal ramus
of spinal nerve

Spinal cord

A

Sympathetic
rami

Body of vertebra

Ventral ramus
of spinal nerve

P

R — L

A

In the illustration above, notice that ventral and dorsal roots join to form a spinal nerve. The spinal nerve then splits into a dorsal *ramus* (plural, *rami*) and a ventral *ramus*. The ventral ramus communicates with a chain of sympathetic (autonomic) ganglia via a pair of thin sympathetic rami. **A,** Superior view of a pair of thoracic spinal nerves.

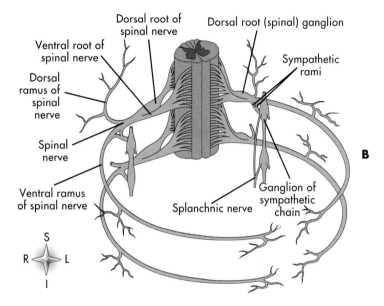

B, Anterior view of several pairs of thoracic spinal nerves.

Spinal Nerves and Peripheral Branches

Spinal Nerves	Plexuses Formed From Anterior Rami	Spinal Nerve Branches From Plexuses	Parts Supplied
CERVICAL			
1		Lesser occipital	Sensory to back of head, front of neck, and upper part of shoulder; motor to numerous neck muscles
2	Cervical plexus	Greater auricular	
3		Cutaneous nerve of neck	
4		Supraclavicular nerves	
		Branches to muscles	
		Phrenic nerve	Diaphragm
CERVICAL		Suprascapular and dorsoscapular	Superficial muscles* of scapula
5		Thoracic nerves, medial and lateral branches	Pectoralis major and minor
6		Long thoracic nerve	Serratus anterior
7	Brachial plexus	Thoracodorsal	Latissimus dorsi
8		Subscapular	Subscapular and teres major muscles
		Axillary (circumflex)	Deltoid and teres minor muscles and skin over deltoid
THORACIC (OR DORSAL)		Musculocutaneous	Muscles of front of arm (biceps brachii, coracobrachialis, and brachialis) and skin on outer side of forearm
1			
2			
3			

	Nerve	Function
4	Ulnar	Flexor carpi ulnaris and part of flexor digitorum profundus; some of muscles of hand; sensory to medial side of hand, little finger, and medial half of fourth finger
5	Median	Rest of muscles of front of forearm and hand; sensory to skin of palmar surface of thumb, index, and middle fingers
6	Radial	Triceps muscle and muscles of back of forearm; sensory to skin of back of forearm and hand
7	Medial cutaneous	Sensory to inner surface of arm and forearm
8		
9	No plexus formed; branches run directly to intercostal muscles and skin of thorax	
10		
11		
12		
LUMBAR		
1	Iliohypogastric ⎫ Sometimes fused	Sensory to anterior abdominal wall
2	Ilioinguinal ⎭	Sensory to anterior abdominal wall and external genitalia; motor to muscles of abdominal wall
2	Genitofemoral	Sensory to skin of external genitalia and inguinal region
4	Lateral femoral cutaneous	Sensory to outer side of thigh
5		

*Although nerves to muscles are considered motor, they do contain some sensory fibers that transmit proprioceptive impulses.

†Sensory fibers from the tibial and peroneal nerves unite to form the medial cutaneous (or sural) nerve that supplies the calf of the leg and the lateral surface of the foot. In the thigh the tibial and common peroneal nerves are usually enclosed in a single sheath to form the *sciatic nerve*, the largest nerve in the body with a width of approximately ¾ of an inch (2 cm). About two thirds of the way down the posterior part of the thigh, it divides into its component parts. Branches of the sciatic nerve extend into the hamstring muscles.

Continued

Spinal Nerves and Peripheral Branches—cont'd

Spinal Nerves	Plexuses Formed From Anterior Rami	Spinal Nerve Branches From Plexuses	Parts Supplied
SACRAL 1 2 3 4 5	Lumbosacral plexus	Femoral	Motor to quadriceps, sartorius, and iliacus muscles; sensory to front of thigh and medial side of lower leg (saphenous nerve)
		Obturator	Motor to adductor muscles of thigh
		Tibial† (medial popliteal)	Motor to muscles of calf of leg; sensory to skin of calf of leg and sole of foot
		Common peroneal (lateral popliteal)	Motor to evertors and dorsiflexors of foot; sensory to lateral surface of leg and dorsal surface of foot
		Nerves to hamstring muscles	Motor to muscles of back of thigh
		Gluteal nerves	Motor to buttock muscles and tensor fasciae latae
		Posterior femoral cutaneous	Sensory to skin of buttocks, posterior surface of thigh, and leg
COCCYGEAL 1	Coccygeal plexus	Pudendal nerve	Motor to perineal muscles; sensory to skin of perineum

$\mathcal{D}$ermatome Distribution of Spinal Nerves

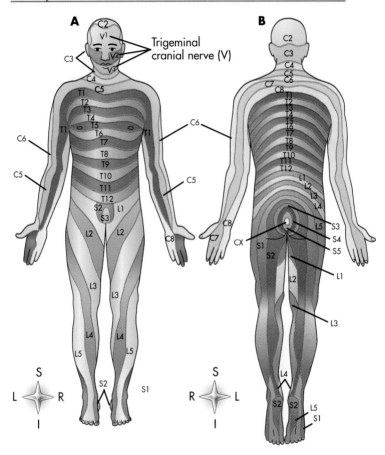

A, The front of the body's surface. **B,** The back of the body's surface. *Continued*

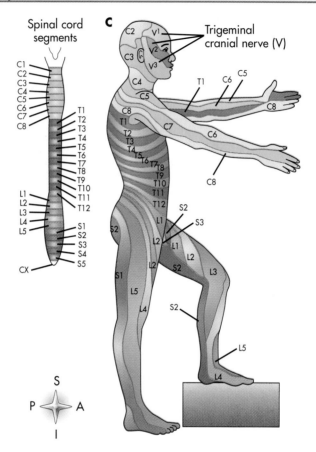

C, The side of the body's surface. The *inset* shows the segments of the spinal cord associated with each of the spinal nerves associated with the sensory dermatomes shown. *C,* Cervical segments and spinal nerves; *T,* thoracic segments and spinal nerves; *L,* lumbar segments and spinal nerves; *S,* sacral segments and spinal nerves.

Cranial Nerves

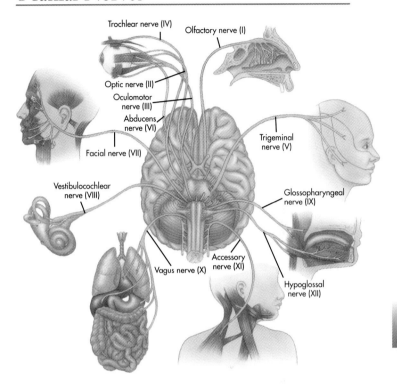

The view of the ventral surface of the brain shows the attachment of the cranial nerves.

Structure and Function of the Cranial Nerves

■ sensory (afferent)
■ motor (efferent)

Nerve	Sensory Fibers			Motor Fibers		Functions
	Receptors	Cell Bodies	Termination	Cell Bodies	Termination	
I OLFACTORY 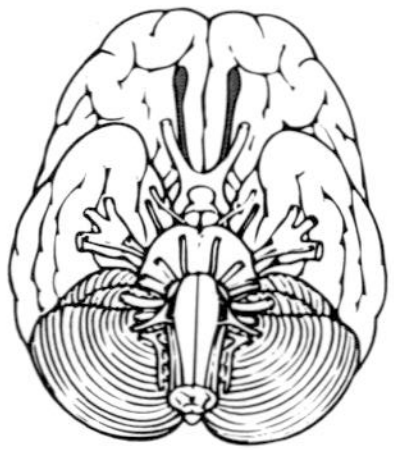	Nasal mucosa	Nasal mucosa	Olfactory bulbs (new relay of neurons to olfactory cortex)			Sense of smell
II OPTIC 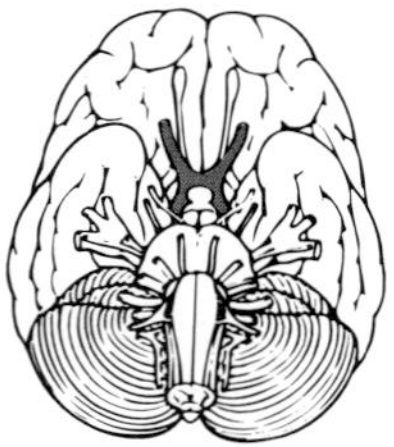	Retina	Retina	Nucleus in thalamus (lateral geniculate); some fibers terminate in superior colliculus of midbrain			Vision

III OCULOMOTOR	External eye muscles except superior oblique and lateral rectus	Trigeminal ganglion	Midbrain (oculomotor nucleus)	Midbrain (oculomotor nucleus)	External eye muscles except superior oblique and lateral rectus; autonomic fibers terminate in ciliary ganglion and then to ciliary and iris muscles	Eye movements, regulation of size of pupil, accommodation (for near vision), proprioception (muscle sense)
IV TROCHLEAR	Superior oblique (proprioceptive)	Trigeminal ganglion	Midbrain	Midbrain	Superior oblique muscle of eye	Eye movements, proprioception

Continued

Structure and Function of the Cranial Nerves—cont'd

■ sensory (afferent)
■ motor (efferent)

| Nerve | Sensory Fibers | | | Motor Fibers | | | Functions |
	Receptors	Cell Bodies	Termination	Cell Bodies	Termination		
V Trigeminal	Skin and mucosa of head, teeth	Trigeminal ganglion	Pons (sensory nucleus)	Pons (motor nucleus)	Muscles of mastication	Sensations of head and face, chewing movements, proprioception
VI Abducens	Lateral rectus (proprioceptive)	Trigeminal ganglion	Pons	Pons	Lateral rectus muscle of eye	Abduction of eye, proprioception

VII FACIAL	Taste buds of anterior two thirds of tongue	Geniculate ganglion	Medulla (nucleus solitarius)	Pons	Superficial muscles of face and scalp; autonomic fibers to salivary and lacrimal glands	Facial expressions, secretion of saliva and tears, taste
VIII VESTIBULOCOCHLEAR						
Vestibular branch	Semicircular canals and vestibule (utricle and saccule)	Vestibular ganglion	Pons and medulla (vestibular nuclei)			Balance or equilibrium sense
Cochlear or auditory branch	Organ of Corti in cochlear duct	Spiral ganglion	Pons and medulla (cochlear nuclei)			Hearing

Continued

Structure and Function of the Cranial Nerves—cont'd

■ sensory (afferent)
■ motor (efferent)

| Nerve | Sensory Fibers | | | Motor Fibers | | | Functions |
	Receptors	Cell Bodies	Termination	Cell Bodies	Termination		
IX GLOSSO-PHARYNGEAL	Pharynx; taste buds and other receptors of posterior one third of tongue	Jugular and petrous ganglia	Medulla (nucleus solitarius)	Medulla (nucleus ambiguus)	Muscles of pharynx		Sensations of tongue, swallowing movements, secretion of saliva, aid in reflex control of blood pressure and respiration
	Carotid sinus and carotid body	Jugular and petrous ganglia	Medulla (respiratory and vasomotor centers)	Medulla at junction of pons (nucleus salivatorius)	Otic ganglion and then to parotid salivary gland		

X VAGUS	Pharynx, larynx, carotid body, and thoracic and abdominal viscera	Jugular and nodose ganglia	Medulla (nucleus solitarius), pons (nucleus of fifth cranial nerve)	Medulla (dorsal motor nucleus)	Ganglia of vagal plexus and then to muscles of pharynx, larynx, and autonomic fibers to thoracic and abdominal viscera	Sensations and movements of organs supplied; (e.g., slows heart, increases peristalsis, and contracts muscles for voice production)

Continued

Structure and Function of the Cranial Nerves—cont'd

■ sensory (afferent)
■ motor (efferent)

Nerve	Sensory Fibers			Motor Fibers			Functions
	Receptors	Cell Bodies	Termination	Cell Bodies	Termination		
XI ACCESSORY	Trapezius and sternocleido-mastoid (proprio-ceptive)	Upper, cervical ganglia	Spinal cord	Medulla (dorsal motor nucleus of vagus and nucleus ambiguus)	Muscles of thoracic and abdominal viscera (autonomic) and pharynx and larynx		Shoulder movements, turning move-ments of head, movements of viscera, voice production, proprioception
				Anterior gray column of first five or six cervical segments of spinal cord	Trapezius and sternocleido-mastoid muscle		

XII HYPOGLOSSAL 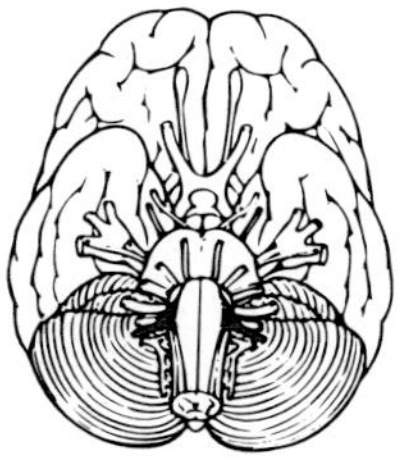	Tongue muscles (proprioceptive)	Trigeminal ganglion	Medulla (hypoglossal nucleus)	Medulla (hypoglossal nucleus)	Muscles of tongue and throat	Tongue movements, proprioception

Autonomic Effector Tissues and Organs

Cardiac Muscle	Smooth Muscle	Glandular Epithelium
Heart	Blood vessels	Sweat glands
	Bronchial tubes	Lacrimal glands
	Stomach	Digestive glands (salivary
	Gallbladder	gastric, pancreas, liver)
	Intestines	Adrenal medulla
	Urinary bladder	
	Spleen	
	Eye (iris and ciliary	
	muscles)	
	Hair follicles	

Autonomic Conduction Paths

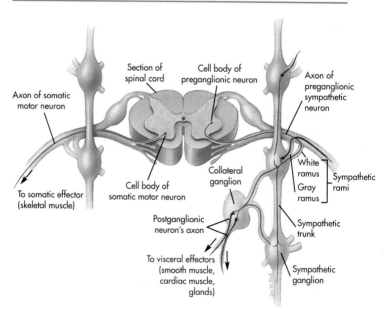

The *left side of the diagram* above shows that one somatic motor neuron conducts impulses all the way from the spinal cord to a somatic effector. Conduction from the spinal cord to any visceral effector, however, requires a relay of at least two autonomic motor neurons—a preganglionic and a postganglionic neuron, shown on the *right side of the diagram.*

Comparison of Somatic Motor and Autonomic Pathways

Feature	Somatic Motor Pathways	Autonomic Efferent Pathways
Direction of information flow	Efferent	Efferent
Number of neurons between CN and effector	One (somatic motor neuron)	Two (preganglionic and postganglionic)
Myelin sheath present	Yes	Preganglionic: yes Postganglionic: no
Location of peripheral fibers	Most cranial nerves and all spinal nerves	Most cranial nerves and all spinal nerves
Effector innervated	Skeletal muscle (voluntary)	Smooth and cardiac muscle, glands (involuntary)
Neurotransmitter	Acetylcholine	Acetylcholine or norepinephrine

Major Autonomic Pathways

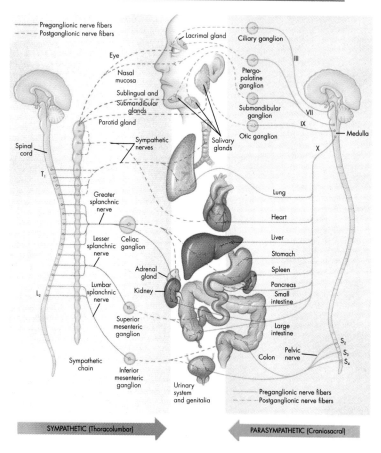

SYMPATHETIC (Thoracolumbar)

PARASYMPATHETIC (Craniosacral)

Comparison of Structural Features of the Sympathetic and Parasympathetic Pathways

Neurons	Sympathetic	Parasympathetic
PREGANGLIONIC NEURONS		
Dendrites and cell bodies	In lateral gray columns of thoracic and first four lumbar segments of spinal cord	In nuclei of brainstem and in lateral gray columns of sacral segments of cord
Axons	In anterior roots of spinal nerves to spinal nerves (thoracic and first four lumbar), to and through white rami to terminate in sympathetic ganglia at various levels or to extend through sympathetic ganglia, to and through splanchnic nerves to terminate in collateral ganglia	From brainstem nuclei through cranial nerve III to ciliary ganglion From nuclei in pons through cranial nerve VII to sphenopalatine or submaxillary ganglion From nuclei in medulla through cranial nerve IX to otic ganglion or through cranial nerves X and XI to cardiac and celiac ganglia, respectively
Distribution	Short fibers from CNS to ganglion	Long fibers from CNS to ganglion
Neurotransmitter	Acetylcholine	Acetylcholine
GANGLIA	Sympathetic chain ganglia (22 pairs); collateral ganglia (celiac, superior, and inferior mesenteric)	Terminal ganglia (in or near effector)

Continued

Comparison of Structural Features of the Sympathetic and Parasympathetic Pathways—cont'd

Neurons	Sympathetic	Parasympathetic
POSTGANGLIONIC NEURONS		
Dendrites and cell bodies	In sympathetic and collateral ganglia	In parasympathetic ganglia (e.g., ciliary, spheno-palatine, submaxillary, otic, cardiac, celiac) located in or near visceral effector organs
Receptors	Cholinergic (nicotinic)	Cholinergic (nicotinic)
Axons	In autonomic nerves and plexuses that innervate thoracic and abdominal viscera and blood vessels in these cavities	In short nerves to various visceral effector organs
	In gray rami to spinal nerves, to smooth muscle of skin blood vessels and hair follicles, and to sweat glands	
Distribution	Long fibers from ganglion to widespread effectors	Short fibers from ganglion to single effector
Neurotransmitter	Norepinephrine (many); acetylcholine (few)	Acetylcholine

£ocations of Neurotransmitters and Receptors of the Autonomic Nervous System

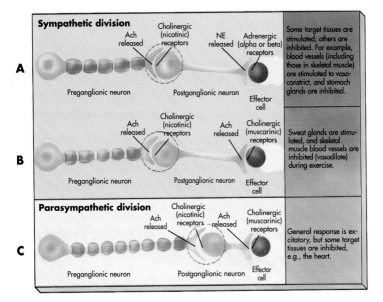

In all pathways, preganglionic fibers are cholinergic, secreting acetylcholine (*Ach*), which stimulates nicotinic receptors in the postganglionic neuron. Most sympathetic postganglionic fibers are adrenergic **(A),** secreting norepinephrine (*NE*), thus stimulating alpha or beta adrenergic receptors. A few sympathetic postganglionic fibers are cholinergic, stimulating muscarinic receptors in effector cells **(B).** All parasympathetic postganglionic fibers are cholinergic **(C),** stimulating muscarinic receptors in effector cells.

Functions of Autonomic Neurotransmitters and Receptors

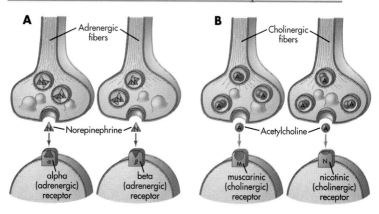

A, Norepinephrine released from adrenergic fibers binds to alpha or beta adrenergic receptors according to the lock-and-key model to produce regulatory effects in the postsynaptic cell. **B,** Acetylcholine released from cholinergic fibers similarly binds to muscarinic or nicotinic cholinergic receptors to produce postsynaptic regulatory effects.

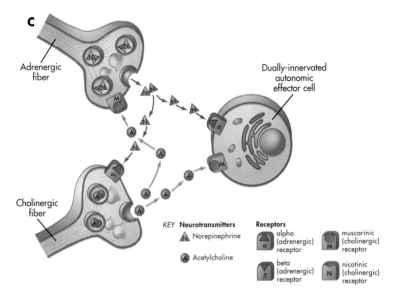

C

Adrenergic fiber

Dually-innervated autonomic effector cell

Cholinergic fiber

KEY **Neurotransmitters**
△ Norepinephrine
Ⓐ Acetylcholine

Receptors
alpha (adrenergic) receptor
beta (adrenergic) receptor
muscarinic (cholinergic) receptor
nicotinic (cholinergic) receptor

C, The complex manner in which neurotransmitters and receptors regulate dually innervated effector cells shows that a summation of effects on receptors at both pre- and postsynaptic locations may occur. For example, norepinephrine released by an adrenergic fiber may bind to postsynaptic alpha (or beta) receptors to influence the effector cell and may also bind to presynaptic alpha (α_2) receptors in a cholinergic fiber to inhibit the release of ACh, a possible antagonist to norepinephrine.

Autonomic Functions

Autonomic Effector	Effect of Sympathetic Stimulation (Neurotransmitter: Norepinephrine Unless Otherwise Stated)	Effect of Parasympathetic Stimulation (Neurotransmitter: Acetylcholine)
CARDIAC MUSCLE	Increased rate and strength of contraction (beta receptors)	Decreased rate and strength of contraction
SMOOTH MUSCLE OF BLOOD VESSELS		
Skin blood vessels	Constriction (alpha receptors)	No effect
Skeletal muscle blood vessels	Dilation (beta receptors)	No effect
Coronary blood vessels	Constriction (alpha receptors)	Dilation
	Dilation (beta receptors)	
Abdominal blood vessels	Constriction (alpha receptors)	No effect
Blood vessels of external genitals	Constriction (alpha receptors)	Dilation of blood vessels causing erection
SMOOTH MUSCLE OF HOLLOW ORGANS AND SPHINCTERS		
Bronchioles	Dilation (beta receptors)	Constriction
Digestive tract, except sphincters	Decreased peristalsis (beta receptors)	Increased peristalsis
Sphincters of digestive tract	Constriction (alpha receptors)	Relaxation
Urinary bladder	Relaxation (beta receptors)	Contraction
Urinary sphincters	Constriction (alpha receptors)	Relaxation
Reproductive ducts	Contraction (alpha receptors)	Relaxation

Eye		
Iris	Contraction of radial muscle; dilated pupil	Contraction of circular muscle; constricted pupil
Ciliary	Relaxation; accommodates for far vision	Contraction; accommodates for near vision
Hairs (pilomotor muscles)	Contraction produces goose pimples, or piloerection (alpha receptors)	No effect
GLANDS		
Sweat	Increased sweat (neurotransmitter, acetylcholine)	No effect
Lacrimal	No effect	Increased secretion of tears
Digestive (salivary, gastric, etc.)	Decreased secretion of saliva; not known for others	Increased secretion of saliva
Pancreas, including islets	Decreased secretion	Increased secretion of pancreatic juice and insulin
Liver	Increased glycogenolysis (beta receptors); increased blood sugar level	No effect
Adrenal medulla*	Increased epinephrine secretion	No effect

*Sympathetic preganglionic axons terminate in contact with secreting cells of the adrenal medulla. Thus the adrenal medulla functions, to quote someone's descriptive phrase, as a "giant sympathetic postganglionic neuron."

*S*ummary of the Sympathetic "Fight-or-Flight" Reaction

Response	Role in Promoting Energy Use by Skeletal Muscles
Increased heart rate	Increased rate of blood flow, thus increased delivery of oxygen and glucose to skeletal muscles
Increased strength of cardiac muscle contraction	Increased rate of blood flow, thus increased delivery of oxygen and glucose to skeletal muscles
Dilation of coronary vessels of the heart	Increased delivery of oxygen and nutrients to cardiac muscle to sustain increased rate and strength of heart contractions
Dilation of blood vessels in skeletal muscles	Increased delivery of oxygen and nutrients to skeletal muscles
Constriction of blood vessels in digestive and other organs	Shunting of blood to skeletal muscles to increase oxygen and glucose delivery
Contraction of spleen and other blood reservoirs	More blood discharged into general circulation, causing increased delivery of oxygen and glucose to skeletal muscles
Dilation of respiratory airways	Increased loading of oxygen into blood
Increased rate and depth of breathing	Increased loading of oxygen into blood
Increased sweating	Increased dissipation of heat generated by skeletal muscle activity
Increased conversion of glycogen into glucose	Increased amount of glucose available to skeletal muscles

Referred Pain

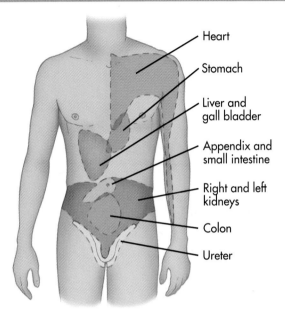

Heart

Stomach

Liver and gall bladder

Appendix and small intestine

Right and left kidneys

Colon

Ureter

The pain resulting from stimulation of nociceptors in deep struc-tures is frequently referred to surface areas. *Referred pain* is the term for this phenomenon. Pain originating in the viscera and other deep structures is generally interpreted as coming from the skin area whose sensory fibers enter the same segment of the spinal cord as the sensory fibers from the deep structure. For example, sensory fibers from the heart enter the first to fourth thoracic segments, and so do sensory fibers from the skin areas over the heart and on the inner surface of the left arm. Pain originating in the heart is referred to those skin areas, but the reason for this is not clear.

Somatic Sensory Receptors

Classification by Structure	By Location and Type	By Activation Stimulus	By Sensation or Function
FREE NERVE ENDINGS			
Nociceptors	Both exteroceptors and visceroceptors—most body tissues	Almost any noxious stimulus; temperature change; mechanical	Pain; temperature; itch; tickle; stretching
Merkel discs	Exteroceptors	Light pressure; mechanical	Discriminative touch
Root hair plexuses	Exteroceptors	Hair movement; mechanical	Sense of "deflection" type movement of hair
ENCAPSULATED NERVE ENDINGS			
Touch and pressure receptors			
Meissner's corpuscle	Exteroceptors; epidermis, hairless skin	Light pressure; mechanical	Discriminative touch; low-frequency vibration
Krause's corpuscle	Mucous membranes	Mechanical; thermal?	Touch; low-frequency vibration; cold?
Ruffini's corpuscle	Dermis of skin, exteroceptors	Mechanical; thermal?	Crude and persistent touch; heat?
Pacinian corpuscle	Dermis of skin, joint capsules	Deep pressure, mechanical	Deep pressure; high-frequency vibration; stretch
Stretch receptors			
Muscle spindles	Skeletal muscle	Stretch, mechanical	Sense of muscle length
Golgi tendon receptors	Musculotendinous junction	Force of contraction and tendon stretch, mechanical	Sense of muscle tension

Olfaction

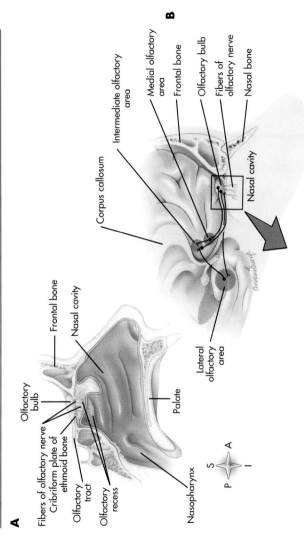

A

Fibers of olfactory nerve
Cribriform plate of ethmoid bone
Olfactory bulb
Olfactory tract
Olfactory recess
Frontal bone
Nasal cavity
Palate
Nasopharynx

B

Intermediate olfactory area
Corpus callosum
Medial olfactory area
Frontal bone
Olfactory bulb
Fibers of olfactory nerve
Nasal bone
Nasal cavity
Lateral olfactory area

Location of olfactory epithelium, olfactory bulb, and neuronal pathways involved in olfaction. **A,** Midsagittal section of the nasal area shows the locations of major olfactory sensory structures. **B,** Major olfactory integration centers of the brain.

Continued

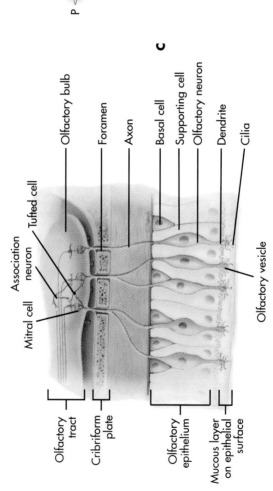

C, Details of the olfactory bulb and olfactory epithelium.

The Tongue

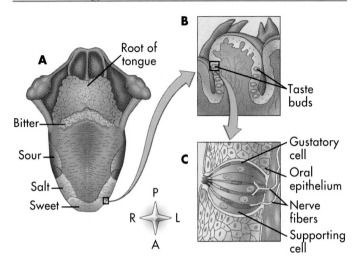

A, Dorsal surface and regions sensitive to various tastes. **B,** Section through a papilla with taste buds on the side. **C,** Enlarged view of a section through a taste bud.

*T*he Ear

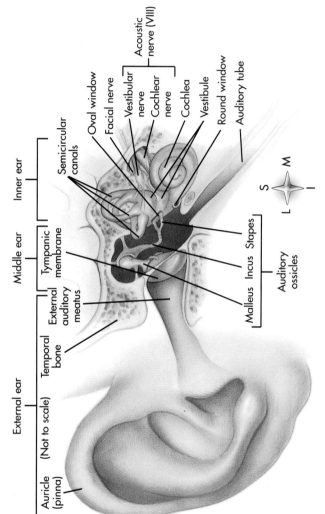

External, middle, and inner ears. *(Anatomic structures are not drawn to scale.)*

The Inner Ear

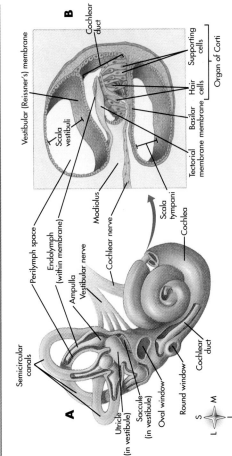

A, The bony labyrinth (*orange*) is the hard outer wall of the entire inner ear and includes semicircular canals, vestibule, and cochlea. Within the bony labyrinth is the membranous labyrinth (*purple*), which is surrounded by perilymph and filled with endolymph. Each ampulla in the vestibule contains a crista ampullaris that detects changes in head position and sends sensory impulses through the vestibular nerve to the brain. **B,** The *inset* shows a section of the membranous cochlea. Hair cells in the organ of Corti detect sound and send the information through the cochlear nerve. The vestibular and cochlear nerves join to form the eighth cranial nerve.

*E*ffect of Sound Waves on Cochlear Structures

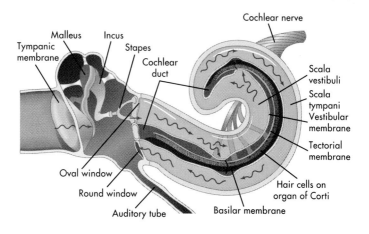

Sound waves strike the tympanic membrane and cause it to vibrate. This causes the membrane of the oval window to vibrate, which causes the perilymph in the bony labyrinth of the cochlea and the endolymph in the membranous labyrinth of the cochlea, or cochlear duct, to move. This movement of endolymph causes the basilar membrane to vibrate, which, in turn, stimulates hair cells on the organ of Corti to transmit nerve impulses along the cranial nerve. Eventually, nerve impulses reach the auditory cortex and are interpreted as sound.

The Macula

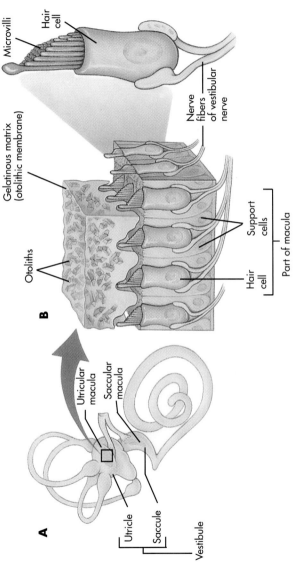

A, Structure of vestibule showing placement of utricular and saccular maculas. **B,** Section of macula showing otoliths.

Continued

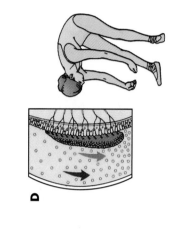

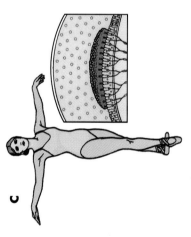

C, Macula stationary in upright position. **D,** Macula displaced by gravity as person bends over.

Structure and Function of the Crista Ampullaris

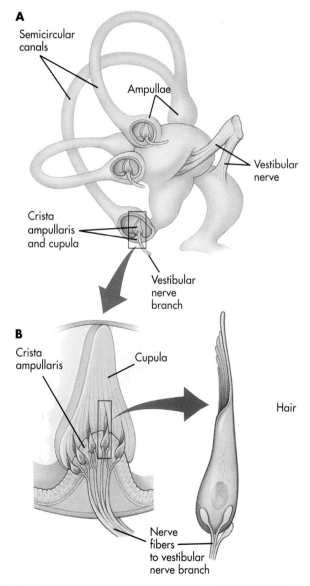

A, Semicircular canals showing location of the crista ampullaris in ampullae. **B,** Enlargement of crista ampullaris and cupula.

Continued

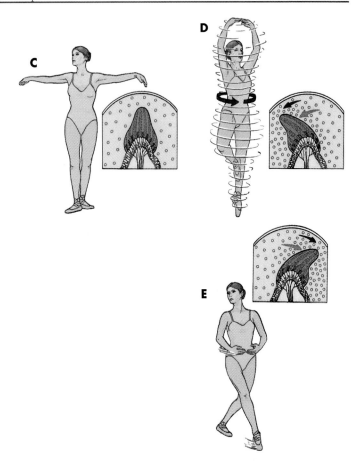

C, When a person is at rest, the crista ampullaris is displaced by the endolymph in a direction opposite to the direction of spin. **D,** As a person begins to spin, the crista ampullaris is displaced (pushed) by the endolymph (fluid inside the canals) in a direction opposite to the direction of spin. Bending of the sensory nerves in a certain direction causes a response that is eventually interpreted in the brain as turning movement in the opposite direction. **E,** As a person stops spinning, the endlymph tends to displace the crista ampullaris in the reverse direction, signaling the brain that turning is slowing or stopping.

The Eyeball

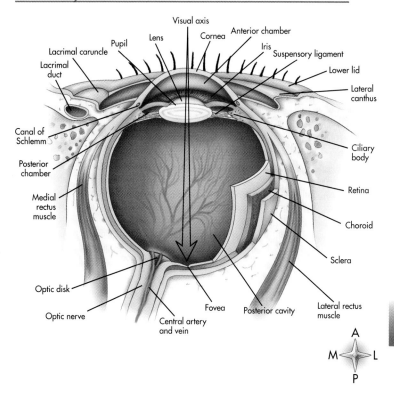

Horizontal section through the left eyeball as viewed from above.

*C*ell Layers of the Retina

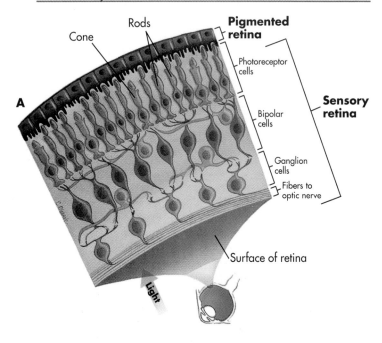

A

Cone

Rods

Pigmented retina

Photoreceptor cells

Bipolar cells

Ganglion cells

Fibers to optic nerve

Sensory retina

Surface of retina

Light

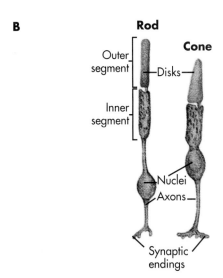

B

Rod

Cone

Outer segment

Disks

Inner segment

Nuclei

Axons

Synaptic endings

A, Pigmented and sensory layers of the retina. **B,** Rod and cone cells. Note their variation in the general structure of a neuron.

Coats of the Eyeball

Location	Posterior Portion	Anterior Portion	Characteristics
Outer coat (sclera)	Sclera proper	Cornea	Protective fibrous coat, cornea transparent, rest of coat white and opaque
Middle coat (choroid)	Choroid proper	Ciliary body, suspensory ligament, iris (pupil is hole in iris); lens suspended in suspensory ligament	Vascular, pigmented coat
Inner coat (retina)	Retina	No anterior portion	Nervous tissue; rods and cones (receptors for second cranial nerve) located in retina

Ophthalmoscopic View of the Retina

Fovea centralis   Macula lutea

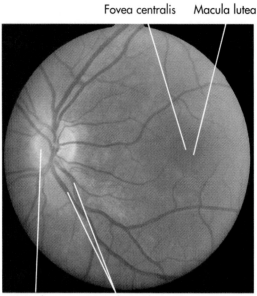

Optic disc   Retinal vessels

This is a view of the retina as seen through the pupil. Note how blood vessels enter the eye through the optic disc (blind spot). Fovea centralis and macula lutea are visible.

Cavities of the Eye

Cavity	Divisions	Location	Contents
Anterior	Anterior chamber	Anterior to iris and posterior to cornea	Aqueous humor
	Posterior chamber	Posterior to iris and anterior to lens	Aqueous humor
Posterior	None	Posterior to lens	Vitreous humor

*E*xtrinsic Muscles of the Eye

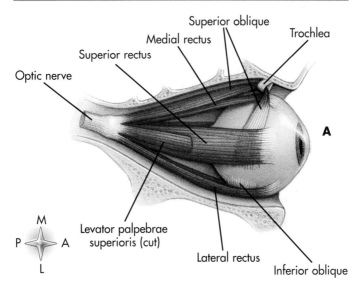

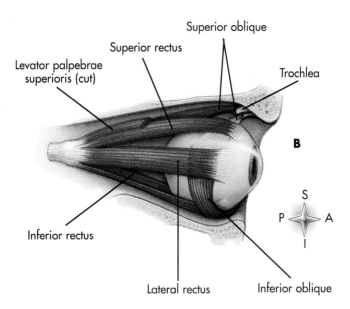

A, Superior view of the right eye showing the extrinsic muscles.
B, Lateral view of the right eye showing the extrinsic muscles.

Accessory Structures of the Eye

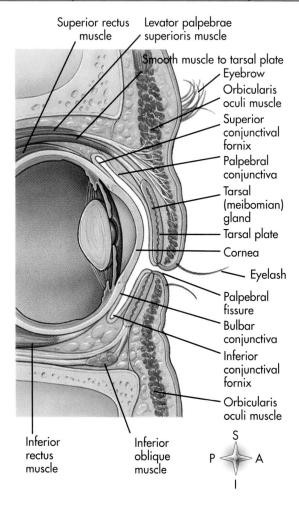

Superior rectus muscle

Levator palpebrae superioris muscle

Smooth muscle to tarsal plate

Eyebrow

Orbicularis oculi muscle

Superior conjunctival fornix

Palpebral conjunctiva

Tarsal (meibomian) gland

Tarsal plate

Cornea

Eyelash

Palpebral fissure

Bulbar conjunctiva

Inferior conjunctival fornix

Orbicularis oculi muscle

Inferior rectus muscle

Inferior oblique muscle

S

P — A

I

Lateral view of the eye with the eyelids closed.

*L*acrimal Apparatus

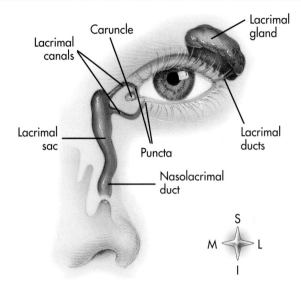

Caruncle

Lacrimal gland

Lacrimal canals

Lacrimal sac

Puncta

Lacrimal ducts

Nasolacrimal duct

S

M ← → L

I

Fluid produced by lacrimal glands (tears) streams across the eye surface, enters the canals, and then passes through the nasolacrimal duct to enter the nose.

*V*isual Fields and Neuronal Pathways of the Eye

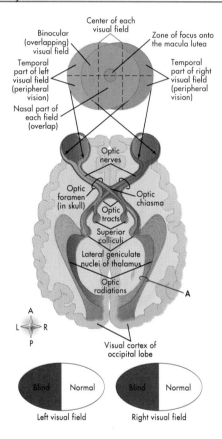

Note in the above illustration the structures that make up each pathway: optic chiasma, lateral geniculate body of thalamus, optic radiations, and visual cortex of occipital lobe. Fibers from the nasal portion of each retina cross over to opposite side at the optic chiasma and terminate in the lateral geniculate nuclei. Location of a lesion in the visual pathway determines the resulting visual defect. Damage at *point A*, for example, would cause blindness in the right nasal and left temporal visual fields, as the ovals beneath indicate. (Trace the visual pathway from *point A* back to the visual field map to see why this is so.) What would be the effect of pressure on the optic chiasma—by a pituitary tumor, for instance? (*Answer.* It would produce blindness in both temporal visual fields. Why? Because it destroys fibers from the nasal side of both retinas.)

9

Endocrine System

The endocrine system and nervous system may work alone or in concert with others as a single neuroendocrine system, performing the same general functions within the body: communication, integration, and control. Both the endocrine system and the nervous system perform their regulatory functions by means of chemical messengers sent to specific cells.

Comparison of Features of the Endocrine System and Nervous System

Feature	Endocrine System	Nervous System
OVERALL FUNCTION	Regulation of effectors to maintain homeostasis	Regulation of effectors to maintain homeostasis
Control by regulatory feedback loops	Yes (endocrine reflexes)	Yes (nervous reflexes)
Effector tissues	Endocrine effectors: virtually all tissues	Nervous effectors: muscle and glandular tissue only
Effector cells*	Target cells (throughout the body)	Postsynaptic cells (in muscle and glandular tissue only)
CHEMICAL MESSENGER*		
Cells that secrete the chemical messenger	Glandular epithelial cells or neurosecretory cells (modified neurons)	Neurotransmitter
	Hormone	Neurons
Distance traveled (and method of travel) by chemical messenger*	Long (by way of circulating blood)	Short (across a microscopic synapse)
Location of receptor in effector cell	On the plasma membrane or within the cell	On the plasma membrane
Characteristics of regulatory effects*	Slow to appear, long-lasting	Appear rapidly, short-lived

$\mathscr{N}$ames and Locations of the Major Endocrine Glands

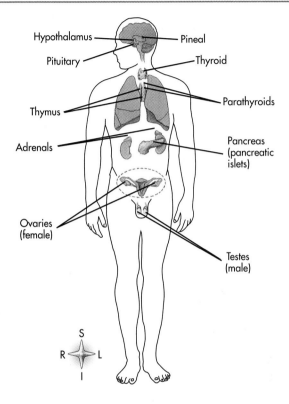

Name	Location
Hypothalamus	Cranial cavity (brain)
Pituitary gland (hypophysis cerebri)	Cranial cavity
Pineal gland	Cranial cavity (brain)
Thyroid gland	Neck
Parathyroid glands	Neck
Thymus	Mediastinum
Adrenal glands	Abdominal cavity (retroperitoneal)
Pancreatic islets	Abdominal cavity (pancreas)
Ovaries	Pelvic cavity
Testes	Scrotum
Placenta	Pregnant uterus

*C*hemical Classification of Hormones

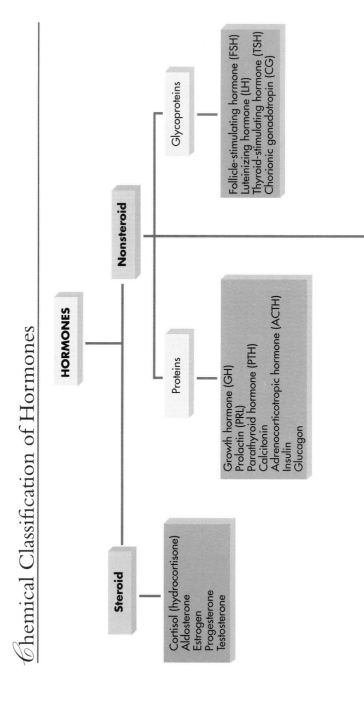

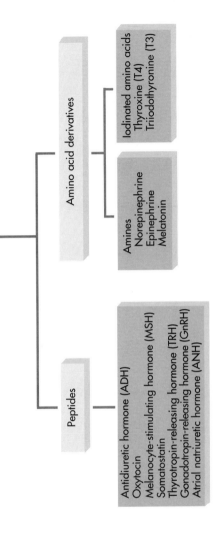

Amino acid derivatives

Iodinated amino acids
Thyroxine (T4)
Triiodothyronine (T3)

Amines
Norepinephrine
Epinephrine
Melatonin

Peptides

Antidiuretic hormone (ADH)
Oxytocin
Melanocyte-stimulating hormone (MSH)
Somatostatin
Thyrotropin-releasing hormone (TRH)
Gonadotropin-releasing hormone (GnRH)
Atrial natriuretic hormone (ANH)

Steroid Hormone Structure

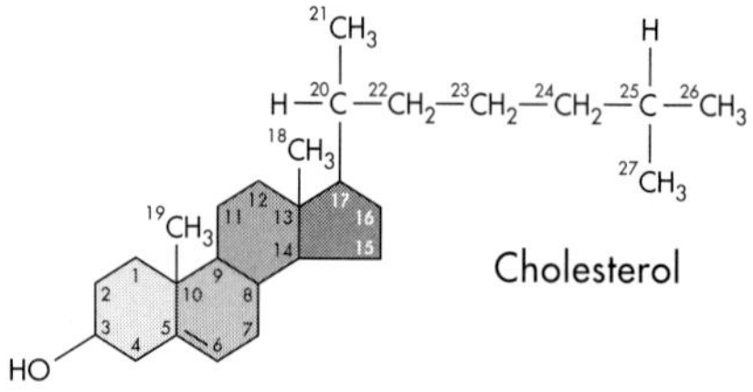

Cholesterol

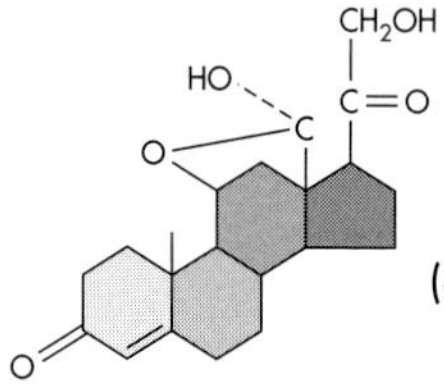

Aldosterone
(a mineralocorticoid)

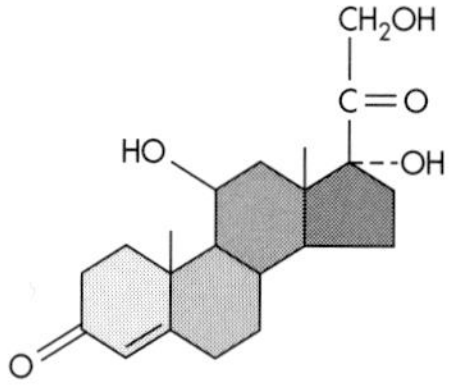

Cortisol
(a glucocorticoid)

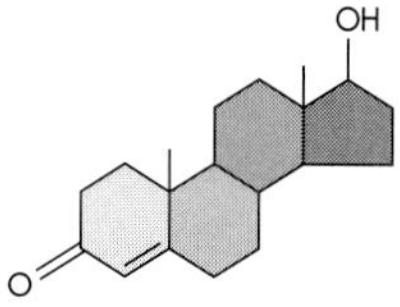

Testosterone
(an androgen)

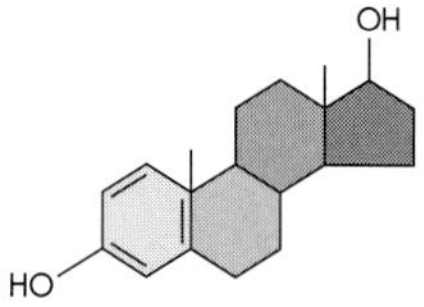

Estradiol
(an estrogen)

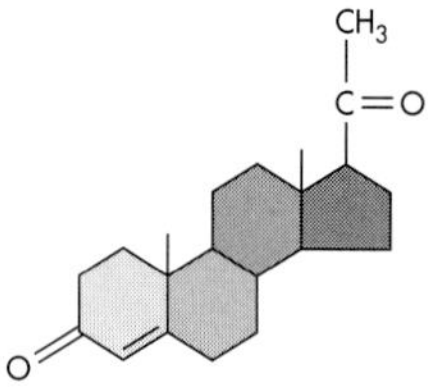

Progesterone

As the examples above show, steroid hormone molecules are very similar in structure to cholesterol (*top*), from which they are all derived.

Nonsteroid Hormone Structure

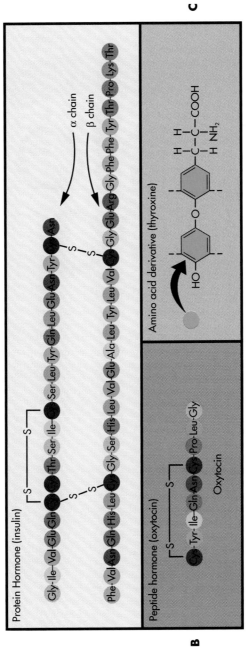

A, Protein hormone molecules are made of long, folded strands of amino acids. **B,** Peptide hormone molecules are smaller strands of amino acids. **C,** Amino acid derivatives are, as their name implies, each derived from a single amino acid.

The Target Cell Concept

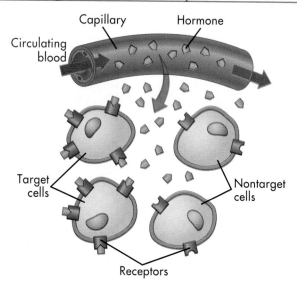

A hormone acts only on cells that have receptors specific to that hormone because the shape of the receptor determines which hormone can react with it. This is an example of the lock-and-key model of biochemical reactions.

Calcium-Calmodulin as a Second Messenger

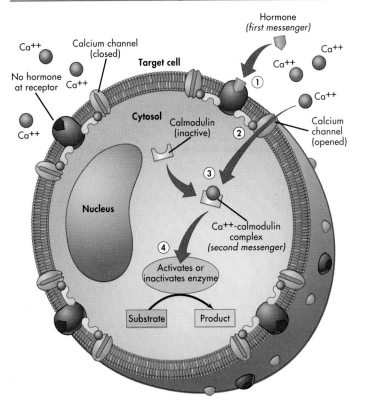

In the above example of a second messenger mechanism, a nonsteroid hormone (first messenger) first binds to a fixed receptor in the plasma membrane (*1*), which activates membrane-bound proteins (G protein and PIP_2) that trigger the opening of calcium channels (*2*). Calcium ions, which are normally at a higher concentration in the extracellular fluid, diffuse into the cell and bind to a calmodulin molecule (*3*). The Ca^{++}-calmodulin complex thus formed is a second messenger that binds to an enzyme to produce an allosteric effect that promotes or inhibits the enzyme's regulatory effect in the target cell (*4*).

Structure of the Prostaglandin Molecule

Structure of prostaglandin $F_{2\alpha}$ ($PGF_{2\alpha}$), showing the typical 20-carbon unsaturated fatty acid structure with a characteristic 5-carbon ring (highlighted in color).

Location and Structure of the Pituitary Gland (Hypophysis)

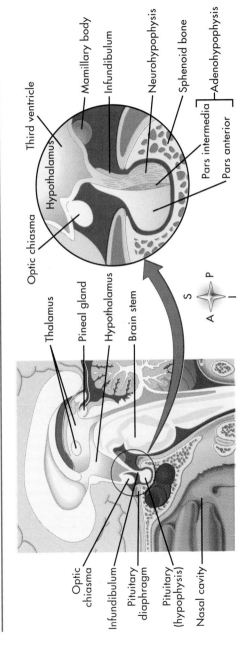

The pituitary gland is located within the sella turcica of the skull's sphenoid bone and is connected to the hypothalamus by a stalklike infundibulum. The infundibulum passes through a gap in the portion of the dura mater that covers the pituitary (the pituitary diaphragm). The *inset* shows that the pituitary is divided into an anterior portion, the adenohypophysis, and a posterior portion, the neurohypophysis. The adenohypophysis is further subdivided into the pars anterior and pars intermedia. The pars intermedia is almost absent in the adult pituitary.

Pituitary Hormones

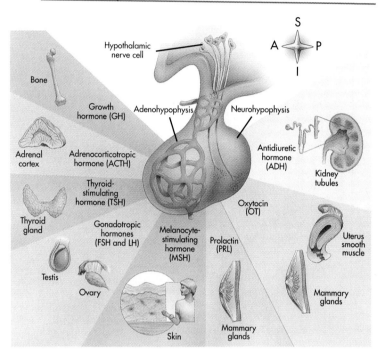

Some of the major hormones of the adenohypophysis and neurohypophysis and their principal target organs.

Hormones of the Hypothalamus

Hormone	Source	Target	Principal Action
Growth hormone–releasing hormone (GRH)	Hypothalamus	Adenohypophysis (somatotrophs)	Stimulates secretion (release) of growth hormone
Growth hormone–inhibiting hormone (GIH), or somatostatin	Hypothalamus	Adenohypophysis (somatotrophs)	Inhibits secretion of growth hormone
Corticotropin-releasing hormone (CRH)	Hypothalamus	Adenohypophysis (corticotrophs)	Stimulates release of adrenocorticotropic hormone (ACTH)
Thyrotropin-releasing hormone (TRH)	Hypothalamus	Adenohypophysis (thyrotrophs)	Stimulates release of thyroid-stimulating hormone (TSH)
Gonadotropin–releasing hormone (GNRH)	Hypothalamus	Adenohypophysis (gonadotrophs)	Stimulates release of gonadotropins (FSH and LH)
Prolactin–releasing hormone (PRH)	Hypothalamus	Adenohypophysis (corticotrophs)	Stimulates secretion of prolactin
Prolactin–inhibiting hormone (PIH)	Hypothalamus	Adenohypophysis (corticotrophs)	Inhibits secretion of prolactin

Thyroid and Parathyroid Glands

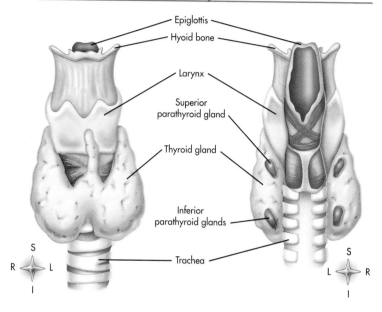

Epiglottis

Hyoid bone

Larynx

Superior parathyroid gland

Thyroid gland

Inferior parathyroid glands

Trachea

$\mathscr{T}$hyroid Gland Tissue

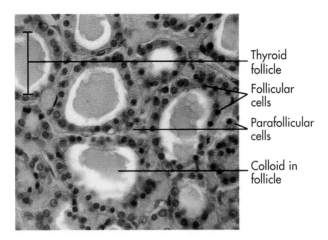

Thyroid
follicle

Follicular
cells

Parafollicular
cells

Colloid in
follicle

Note in the above photomicrograph that each of the follicles is filled with colloid (×140).

Hormones of the Thyroid and Parathyroid Glands

Hormone	Source	Target	Principal Action
Triiodothyronine (T_3)	Thyroid gland (follicular cells)	General	Increases rate of metabolism
Tetraiodothyronine (T_4), or thyroxine	Thyroid gland (follicular cells)	General	Increases rate of metabolism (usually converted to T_3 first)
Calcitonin (CT)	Thyroid gland (parafollicular cells)	Bone tissue	Increases calcium storage in bone, lowering blood Ca^{++} levels
Parathyroid hormone (PTH) or parathormone	Parathyroid glands	Bone tissue and intestinal tract	Increases calcium removal from storage in bone and increases absorption of calcium by intestines, increasing blood Ca^{++} levels

Structure of the Adrenal Gland

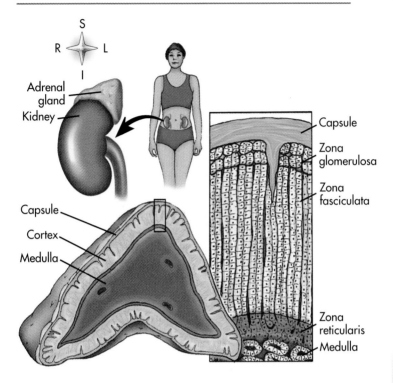

The zona glomerulosa of the cortex secretes aldosterone. The zona fasciculata secretes abundant amounts of glucocorticoids, chiefly cortisol. The zona reticularis secretes minute amounts of sex hormones and glucocorticoids.

Hormones of the Adrenal Glands

Hormone	Source	Target	Principal Action
Aldosterone	Adrenal cortex (zona glomerulosa)	Kidney	Stimulates kidney tubules to conserve sodium, which, in turn, triggers the release of ADH and the resulting conservation of water by the kidney
Cortisol (hydrocortisone)	Adrenal cortex (zona fasciculata)	General	Influences metabolism of food molecules; in large amounts, it has an antiinflammatory effect
Adrenal androgens	Adrenal cortex (zona reticularis)	Sex organs, other effectors	Exact role uncertain, but may support sexual function
Adrenal estrogens	Adrenal cortex (zona reticularis)	Sex organs	Thought to be physiologically insignificant
Epinephrine (adrenaline)	Adrenal medulla	Sympathetic effectors	Enhances and prolongs the effects of the sympathetic division of the autonomic nervous system
Norepinephrine	Adrenal medulla	Sympathetic effectors	Enhances and prolongs the effects of the sympathetic division of the autonomic nervous system

Structure and Location of the Pancreas

The pancreas is an elongated gland weighing up to 100 g (3.5 ounces). The "head" of the gland lies in the C-shaped beginning of the small intestine (duodenum), with its body extending horizontally behind the stomach and its tail touching the spleen. The endocrine portion of the pancreas is composed of both endocrine and exocrine tissues. The endocrine portion is made up of scattered, tiny islands of cells, called pancreatic islets.

*H*ormones of the Pancreatic Islets

Hormone	Source	Target	Principal Action
Glucagon	Pancreatic islets (alpha [α] cells or A cells)	General	Promotes movement of glucose from storage and into the blood
Insulin	Pancreatic islets (beta [β] cells or B cells)	General	Promotes movement of glucose out of the blood and into cells
Somatostatin	Pancreatic islets (delta [δ] cells or D cells)	Pancreatic cells and other effectors	Can have general effects in the body, but primary role seems to be regulation of secretion of other pancreatic hormones
Pancreatic polypeptide	Pancreatic islets (pancreatic polypeptide [PP] or F cells)	Intestinal cells and other effectors	Exact function uncertain, but seems to influence absorption in the digestive tract

Hormones of Other Major Endocrine Glands

Hormone	Source	Target	Principal Action
Testosterone	Testes	Spermatogenic cells; muscle; bone tissue; other tissues	Responsible for growth and maintenance of male sexual characteristics and for sperm production
Estrogen	Ovarian follicles	Uterus; mammary glands; other tissues	Promote the development and maintenance of female sexual characteristics and the proper sequence of events in the female reproductive cycle (menstrual cycle)
Progesterone	Corpus luteum	Uterus; other tissues	Maintains (along with estrogen) the lining of the uterus necessary for successful pregnancy
Human chorionic gonadotropin (hCG)	Chorion (a fetal tissue component of the placenta)	Ovary	Stimulates development and hormone secretion by maternal ovarian tissues

Cardiovascular System

Blood, the complex fluid tissue that serves to transport respiratory gases and key nutrients to cells and carry away wastes, fills the cardiovascular system. Blood is moved through a closed pathway, or circuit, of vessels by the pumping action of the heart.

Composition of Whole Blood

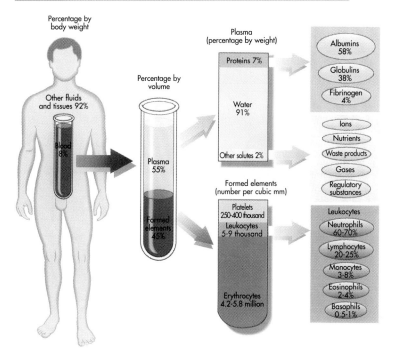

Percentage by body weight

Other fluids and tissues 92%

Blood 8%

Percentage by volume

Plasma 55%

Formed elements 45%

Plasma (percentage by weight)

Proteins 7%

Water 91%

Other solutes 2%

Albumins 58%

Globulins 38%

Fibrinogen 4%

Ions

Nutrients

Waste products

Gases

Regulatory substances

Formed elements (number per cubic mm)

Platelets 250-400 thousand

Leukocytes 5-9 thousand

Erythrocytes 4.2-5.8 million

Leukocytes

Neutrophils 60-70%

Lymphocytes 20-25%

Monocytes 3-8%

Eosinophils 2-4%

Basophils 0.5-1%

This illustration shows approximate values for the components of blood in a normal adult.

Formation of Blood Cells

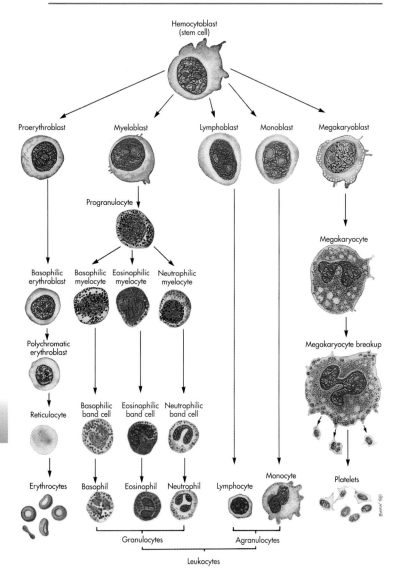

The hematopoietic stem cell serves as the original stem cell from which all formed elements of the blood are derived. Note that all five precursor cells, which ultimately produce the different components of the formed elements, are derived from the hematopoietic stem cell.

Classes of Blood Cells

Cell Type	Description	Function	Life Span
Erythrocyte	7 μm in diameter; concave disk shape; entire cell stains pale pink; no nucleus	Transportation of respiratory gases (O_2 and CO_2)	105 to 120 days
Neutrophil	12–15 μm in diameter; spherical shape; multilobed nucleus; small, pink–purple staining cytoplasmic granules	Cellular defense–phagocytosis of small pathogenic microorganisms	Hours to 3 days
Basophil	11–14 μm in diameter; spherical shape; generally two-lobed nucleus; large purple staining cytoplasmic granules	Secretes heparin (anticoagulant) and histamine (important in inflammatory response)	Hours to 3 days
Eosinophil	10–12 μm in diameter; spherical shape; generally two-lobed nucleus; large orange–red staining cytoplasmic granules	Cellular defense–phagocytosis of large pathogenic microorganisms such as protozoa and parasitic worms; releases antiinflammatory substances in allergic reactions	10 to 12 days
Lymphocyte	6–9 μm in diameter; spherical shape; round (single lobe) nucleus; small lymphocytes have scant cytoplasm	Humoral defense–secretes antibodies; involved in immune system response and regulation	Days to years
Monocyte	12–17 μm in diameter; spherical shape; nucleus generally kidney-bean or "horseshoe" shaped with convoluted surface; ample cytoplasm often "steel blue" in color	Capable of migrating out of the blood to enter tissue spaces as a *macrophage*–an aggressive phagocytic cell capable of ingesting bacteria, cellular debris, and cancerous cells	Months
Platelet	2–5 μm in diameter; irregularly shaped fragments; cytoplasm contains very small pink staining granules	Releases clot activating substances and helps in formation of actual blood clot by forming platelet "plugs"	7 to 10 days

Differential Count of White Blood Cells

| Class | Differential Count* | |
	Normal Range (%)	Typical Value (%)
Neutrophils	65 to 75	65
Eosinophils	2 to 5	3
Basophils	½ to 1	1
Lymphocytes (large and small)	20 to 25	25
Monocytes	3 to 8	6
TOTAL	100	100

*In any differential count the sum of the percentages of the different kinds of WBCs must, of course, total 100%.

Results of Different Combinations of Donor and Recipient Blood

| Recipient's blood | | Reactions with donor's blood | | | |
RBC antigens	Plasma antibodies	Donor type O	Donor type A	Donor type B	Donor type AB
None (Type O)	Anti-A Anti-B				
A (Type A)	Anti-B				
B (Type B)	Anti-A				
AB (Type AB)	(none)				

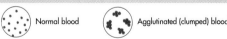

Normal blood   Agglutinated (clumped) blood

The *left columns* show the recipient's blood characteristics, and the *top row* shows the donor's blood type.

Coagulation Factors—Standard Nomenclature and Synonyms

Factor	Common Synonym(s)
Factor I	Fibrinogen
Factor II	Prothrombin
Factor III	Thromboplastin
	Thrombokinase
Factor IV	Calcium
Factor V	Proaccelerin
	Labile factor
Factor VI (now obsolete)	None in use
Factor VII	Serum prothrombin conversion accelerator (SPCA)
Factor VIII	Antihemophilic globulin (AHG)
	Antihemophilic factor (AHF)
Factor IX	Plasma thromboplastin component (PTC), Christmas factor
Factor X	Stuart factor
Factor XI	Plasma thromboplastin antecedent (PTA)
Factor XII	Hageman factor
Factor XIII	Fibrin-stabilizing factor

Clot Formation

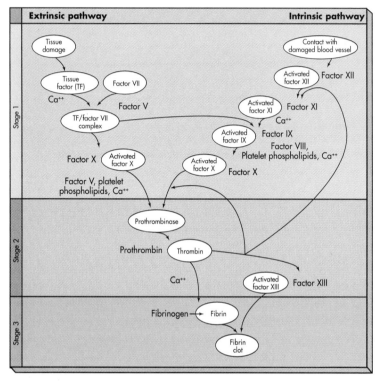

A, Extrinsic clotting pathway. *Stage 1*: Damaged tissue releases tissue factor, which with factor VII and calcium ions activates factor X. Activated factor X, factor V, phospholipids, and calcium ions form prothrombinase. *Stage 2*: Prothrombin is converted to thrombin by prothrombinase. *Stage 3*: Fibrinogen is converted to fibrin by thrombin. Fibrin forms a clot. **B,** Intrinsic clotting pathway. *Stage 1*: Damaged vessels cause activation of factor XII. Activated factor XII activates factor XI, which activates factor IX. Factor IX, along with factor VIII and platelet phospholipids, activates factor X. Activated factor X, factor V, phospholipids, and calcium ions form prothrombinase. *Stages 2 and 3* take the same course as the extrinsic clotting pathway.

Blood, Plasma, and Serum Values

Test	Normal Values*	Significance of a Change
Acid phosphatase	*Women:* 0.01–0.56 sigma U/ml *Men:* 0.13–0.63 sigma U/ml	↑ in prostate cancer ↑ in kidney disease ↑ after trauma and in fever
Alkaline phosphatase	*Adult:* 13–39 IU/l *Child:* up to 104 IU/l	↑ in bone disorders ↑ in liver disease ↑ during pregnancy ↑ in hypothyroidism
Bicarbonate	22–26 mEq/L	↑ in metabolic alkalosis ↑ in respiratory alkalosis ↑ in metabolic acidosis ↑ in respiratory alkalosis
Blood urea nitrogen (BUN)	5–25 mg/100 ml	↑ with increased protein intake ↑ in kidney failure
Blood volume	*Women:* 65 ml/kg body weight *Men:* 69 ml/kg body weight	↓ during hemorrhage
Calcium	8.4–10.5 mg/100 ml	↑ in hypervitaminosis D ↑ in hyperparathyroidism ↑ in bone cancer and other bone diseases ↓ in severe diarrhea ↓ in hypoparathyroidism ↓ in avitaminosis D (rickets and osteomalacia)

Continued

*Values vary with the analysis method used; 100 ml = 1 dl.

$\mathcal{B}$lood, Plasma, and Serum Values—cont'd

Test	Normal Values*	Significance of a Change
Carbon dioxide content	24-32 mEq/L	↑ in severe vomiting ↑ in respiratory disorders ↑ in obstruction of intestines ↓ in acidosis ↓ in severe diarrhea ↓ in kidney disease
Chloride	96-107 mEq/L	↑ in hyperventilation ↑ in kidney disease ↑ in Cushing's syndrome ↓ in diabetic acidosis ↓ in severe diarrhea ↓ in severe burns ↓ in Addison's disease
Clotting time	5-10 minutes	↓ in hemophilia ↓ (occasionally) in other clotting disorders
Copper	100-200 μg/100 ml	↑ in some liver disorders
Creatine phosphokinase (CPK)	*Women:* 5-35 mU/ml *Men:* 5-55 mU/ml	↑ in Duchenne's muscular dystrophy ↑ during myocardial infarction ↑ in muscle trauma
Creatine	0.6-1.5 mg/100 ml	↑ in some kidney disorders

Glucose	70–110 mg/100 ml (fasting)	↑ in diabetes mellitus
		↑ in kidney disease
		↑ in liver disease
		↑ during pregnancy
		↑ in hyperthyroidism
		↓ in hypothyroidism
		↓ in Addison's disease
		↓ in hyperinsulinism
Hematocrit (packed cell volume)	*Women:* 38%–47%	↑ in polycythemia
	Men: 40%–54%	↑ in severe dehydration
		↓ in anemia
		↓ in leukemia
		↓ in hyperthyroidism
		↓ in cirrhosis of liver
Hemoglobin	*Women:* 12–16 g/100 ml	↑ in polycythemia
	Men: 13–18 g/100 ml	↑ in chronic obstructive pulmonary disease
	Newborn: 14–20 g/100 ml	↑ in congestive heart failure
		↓ in anemia
		↓ in hyperthyroidism
		↓ in cirrhosis of liver

*Values vary with the analysis method used; 100 ml = 1 dl.

Continued

Blood, Plasma, and Serum Values—cont'd

Test	Normal Values*	Significance of a Change
Iron	50–150 µg/100 ml (can be higher in men)	↑ in liver disease ↑ in anemia (some forms) ↓ in iron-deficiency anemia
Lactic dehydrogenase (LDH)	60–120 U/ml	↑ during myocardial infarction ↑ in anemia (several forms) ↑ liver disease ↑ in acute leukemia and other cancers
Lipids—total	450–1,000 mg/100 ml	↑ (total) in diabetes mellitus
Cholesterol—total	120–220 mg/100 ml	↑ (total) in kidney disease
High-density lipoprotein (HDL)	>40 mg/100 ml	↑ (total) in hypothyroidism
Low-density lipoprotein (LDL)	<180 mg/100 ml	↓ (total) in hyperthyroidism ↑ in inherited hypercholesterolemia ↑ (cholesterol) in chronic hepatitis
Triglycerides	40–150 mg/100 ml	↓ (cholesterol) in acute hepatitis
Phospholipids	145–200 mg/100 ml	↑ (HDL) with regular exercise
Fatty acids	190–420 mg/100 ml	
Mean corpuscular volume	82–98 µl	↑ or ↓ in various forms of anemia
Osmolality	285–295 mOsm/L	↑ or ↓ in fluid and electrolyte imbalances

P_{CO_2}	35–43 mm Hg	↑ in severe vomiting ↑ in respiratory disorders ↑ in obstruction of intestines ↓ in acidosis ↓ in severe diarrhea ↓ in kidney disease
pH	7.35–7.45	↑ during hyperventilation ↑ in Cushing's syndrome ↓ during hypoventilation ↓ in acidosis ↓ in Addison's disease
Phosphorus	2.5–4.5 mg/100 ml	↑ in hypervitaminosis D ↑ in kidney disease ↑ in hypoparathyroidism ↑ in acromegaly ↓ in hyperparathyroidism ↓ in hypovitaminosis D (rickets and osteomalacia)
Plasma volume	*Women:* 40 ml/kg body weight *Men:* 39 ml/kg body weight	↑ or ↓ in fluid and electrolyte imbalances ↓ during hemorrhage

*Values vary with the analysis method used; 100 ml = 1 dl.

Continued

ℬlood, Plasma, and Serum Values—cont'd

Test	Normal Values*	Significance of a Change
Platelet count	150,000–400,000/mm³	↑ in heart disease
		↑ in cancer
		↑ in cirrhosis of liver
		↑ after trauma
		↓ in anemia (some forms)
		↓ during chemotherapy
		↓ in some allergies
Po₂	75–100 mm Hg (breathing standard air)	↑ in polycythemia
		↓ in anemia
		↓ in chronic obstructive pulmonary disease
Potassium	3.8–5.1 mEq/L	↑ in hypoaldosteronism
		↑ in acute kidney failure
		↓ in vomiting or diarrhea
		↓ in starvation
Protein—total	6–8.4 g/100 ml	↑ (total) in severe dehydration
Albumin	3.5–5 g/100 ml	↓ (total) during hemorrhage
Globulin	2.3–3.5 g/100 ml	↓ (total) in starvation
Red blood cell count	*Women:* 4.2–5.4 million/mm³	↑ in polycythemia
	Men: 4.5–6.2 million/mm³	↑ in dehydration
		↓ in anemia (several forms)
		↓ in Addison's disease
		↓ in systemic lupus erythematosus

Reticulocyte count	25,000–75,000/mm³ (0.5%–1.5% of RBC count)	↑ in hemolytic anemia
		↑ in leukemia and metastatic carcinoma
		↓ in pernicious anemia
		↓ in iron–deficiency anemia
		↓ during radiation therapy
Sodium	136–145 mEq/L	↑ in dehydration
		↑ in trauma or disease of the central nervous system
		↑ or ↓ in kidney disorders
		↓ in excessive sweating, vomiting, diarrhea
		↓ in burns (sodium shift into cells)
Specific gravity	1.058	↑ or ↓ in fluid imbalances
Transaminase	10–40 U/ml	↑ during myocardial infarction
		↑ in liver disease
Uric acid	*Women:* 2.5–7.5 mg/100 ml	↑ in gout
	Men: 3–9 mg/100 ml	↑ in toxemia of pregnancy
		↑ during trauma
Viscosity	1.4–1.8 times the viscosity of water	↑ in polycythemia
		↑ in dehydration

*Values vary with the analysis method used; 100 ml = 1 dl.

Continued

Blood, Plasma, and Serum Values—cont'd

Test	Normal Values*	Significance of a Change
White blood cell count		
Total	4,500-11,000/mm³	↑ (total) in acute infections
Neutrophils	60%-70% of total	↑ (total) in trauma
Eosinophils	2%-4% of total	↑ (total) some cancers
Basophils	0.5%-1% of total	↓ (total) in anemia (some forms)
Lymphocytes	20-25% of total	↓ (total) during chemotherapy
Monocytes	3%-8% of total	↑ (neutrophil) in acute infection
		↑ (eosinophil) in allergies
		↓ (basophil) in severe allergies
		↑ (lymphocyte) during antibody reactions
		↑ (monocyte) in chronic infections

*Values vary with the analysis method used; 100 ml = 1 dl.

Conversion Factors (SI Units)

Component	Normal Range in Units as Customarily Reported	Conversion Factor	Normal Range in SI Units, Molecular Units, International Units, or Decimal Fractions
BIOCHEMICAL COMPONENTS OF BLOOD*			
Acetoacetic acid (S)	0.2–1.0 mg/dL	98	19.6–98.0 μmol/L
Acetone (S)	0.3–2.0 mg/dL	172	51.6–344.0 μmol/L
Albumin (S)	3.2–4.5 g/dL	10	32–45 g/L
Ammonia (P)	20–120 μg/dL	0.588	11.7–70.5 μmol/L
Amylase (S)	60–160 Somogyi units/dL	1.85	111–296 U/L
Base, total (S)	145–160 mEq/L	1	145–160 mmol/L
Bicarbonate (P)	21–28 mEq/L	1	21–28 mmol/L
Bile acids (S)	0.3–3.0 mg/dL	10	3–30 mg/L
		2.547	0.8–7.6 μmol/L
Bilirubin, direct (S)	Up to 0.3 mg/dL	17.1	Up to 5.1 μmol/L
Bilirubin, indirect (S)	0.1–1.0 mg/dL	17.1	1.7–17.1 μmol/L
Blood gases (B)			
P_{CO_2} arterial	35–40 mm Hg	0.133	4.66–5.32 kPa
P_{O_2} arterial	95–100 mm Hg	0.133	12.64–13.30 kPa
Calcium (S)	8.5–10.5 mg/dL	0.25	2.1–2.6 mmol/L
Chloride (S)	95–103 mEq/L	1	95–103 mmol/L
Creatine (S)	0.1–0.4 mg/dL	76.3	7.6–30.5 μmol/L
Creatinine (S)	0.6–1.2 mg/dL	88.4	53–106 μmol/L

*The International Committee for Standardization in Hematology recommends that the numbers remain the same but that the units change, so that hemoglobin is expressed as grams per deciliter (g/dL) even though other measurements are expressed as units per liter (U/L).

Conversion Factors (SI Units)—cont'd

Component	Normal Range in Units as Customarily Reported	Conversion Factor	Normal Range in SI Units, Molecular Units, International Units, or Decimal Fractions
BIOCHEMICAL COMPONENTS OF BLOOD—cont'd			
Creatinine clearance (P)	107–139 mL/min	0.0167	1.78–2.32 mL/s
Fatty acids (total) (S)	8–20 mg/dL	0.01	0.08–2.00 mg/L
Fibrinogen (P)	200–400 mg/dL	0.01	2.00–4.00 g/L
Gamma globulin (S)	0.5–1.6 g/dL	10	5–16 g/L
Globulins (total) (S)	2.3–3.5 q/dL	10	23–35 g/L
Glucose (fasting) (S)	70–110 mg/dL	0.055	3.85–6.05 mmol/L
Insulin (radioimmunoassay) (P)	4.24 μIU/ml	0.0417	0.17–1.00 μg/L
	0.20–0.84 μg/L	172.2	35–145 mol/L
Iodine, BEI (S)	3.5–6.5 μg/dL	0.079	0.28–0.51 μmol/L
Iodine, PBI (S)	4.0–8.0 μg/dL	0.079	0.32–0.63 μmol/L
Iron, total (S)	60–150 μg/dL	0.179	11–27 μmol/L
Iron-binding capacity (S)	300–360 μg/dL	0.179	54–64 μmol/L
17-Ketosteroids (P)	25–125 μg/dL	0.01	0.25–1.25 mg/L
Lactic dehydrogenase (S)	80–120 units at 30° C	0.48	38–62 U/L at 30° C
	Lactate → pyruvate		
	100–190 U/L at 37° C	1	100–190 U/L at 37° C
Lipase (S)	0–1.5 U/ml	278	0–417 U/L
	Cherry–Crandall		

Lipids (total) (S)	400-800 mg/dL	0.01	4.00-8.00 g/L
Cholesterol	150-250 mg/dL	0.026	3.9-6.5 mmol/L
Triglycerides	75-165 mg/dL	0.0114	0.85-1.89 mmol/L
Phospholipids	150-380 mg/dL	0.01	1.50-380 g/L
Free fatty acids	9.0-15.0 mM/L	1	9.0-15.0 mmol/L
Nonprotein nitrogen (S)	20-35 mg/dL	0.714	14.3-25.0 mmol/L
Phosphatase (P)			
Acid (units/dL)			
Cherry-Crandall		2.77	0-5.5 U/L
King-Armstrong		1.77	0-5.5 U/L
Bodansky		5.37	0-5.5 U/L
Alkaline (units/dL)			
King-Armstrong		1.77	30-120 U/L
Bodansky		5.37	30-120 U/L
Bessey-Lowry-Brock		16.67	30-120 U/L
Phosphorus, inorganic (S)	3.0-4.5 mg/dL	0.323	0.97-1.45 mmol/L
Potassium (P)	3.8-5.0 mEq/L	1	3.8-5.0 mmol/L
Proteins, total (S)	6.0-7.8 g/dL	10	60-78 g/L
Albumin	3.2-4.5 g/dL	10	32-45 g/L
Globulin	2.3-3.5 g/dL	10	23-35 g/L
Sodium (P)	136-142 mEq/L	1	136-142 mmol/L

*The International Committee for Standardization in Hematology recommends that the numbers remain the same but that the units change, so that hemoglobin is expressed as grams per deciliter (g/dL) even though other measurements are expressed as units per liter (U/L).

Continued

Conversion Factors (SI Units)—cont'd

Component	Normal Range in Units as Customarily Reported	Conversion Factor	Normal Range in SI Units, Molecular Units, International Units, or Decimal Fractions
BIOCHEMICAL COMPONENTS OF BLOOD—cont'd			
Testosterone: Male (S)	300–1,200 ng/dL	0.035	10.5–42.0 nmol/L
Female	30–95 ng/dL	0.035	1.0–3.3 nmol/L
Thyroid tests (S)			
Thyroxine (T_4)	4–11 µg/dL	12.87	51–142 nmol/L
T_4 expressed as iodine	3.2–7.2 µg/dL	79.0	253–569 nmol/L
T_3 resin uptake	25%–38% relative uptake	0.01	0.25%–0.38% relative uptake
TSH (S)	10 µU/mL	1	$<10^{-3}$ IU/L
Urea nitrogen (S)	8–23 mg/dL	0.357	2.9–82. mmol/L
Uric acid (S)	2–6 mg/dL	59.5	0.120–0.360 mmol/L
Vitamin B_{12} (S)	160–195 pg/mL	0.74	118–703 pmol/L
HEMATOLOGY VALUES*			
Red cell volume (male)	25–35 mL/kg body weight	0.001	0.025–0.035 L/kg body weight
Hematocrit	40%–50%	0.01	0.40–0.50
Hemoglobin	13.5–18.0 g/dL	10	135–180 g/L
Hemoglobin	13.5–18.0 g/dL	0.155	2.09–2.79 mmol/L
RBC count	$4.5–6 \times 10^6/µL$	1	$4.6–6 \times 10^{12}/L$
WBC count	$4.5–10 \times 10^3/µL$	1	$4.5–10 \times 10^9/L$
Mean corpuscular volume	80–96 µm³	1	80–96 fL

*The International Committee for Standardization in Hematology recommends that the numbers remain the same but that the units change, so that hemoglobin is expressed as grams per deciliter (g/dL) even though other measurements are expressed as units per liter (U/L).

The Heart and Great Vessels

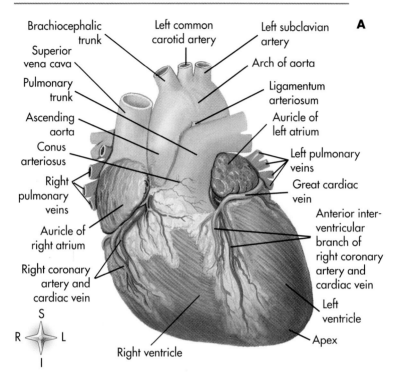

A, Anterior view of the heart and great vessels.

Continued

The Heart and Great Vessels—cont'd

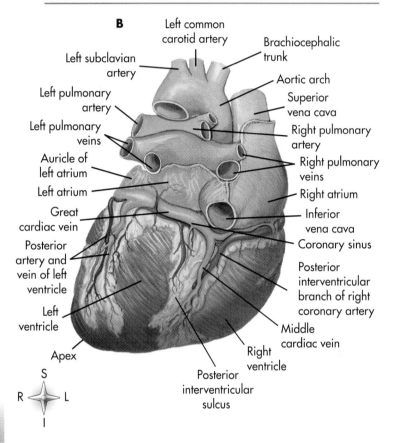

B, Posterior view of the heart and great vessels.

Wall of the Heart

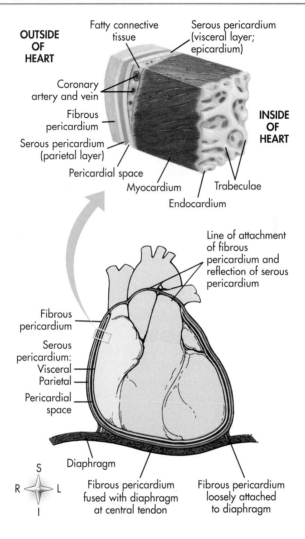

OUTSIDE OF HEART

Fatty connective tissue

Serous pericardium (visceral layer; epicardium)

Coronary artery and vein

Fibrous pericardium

Serous pericardium (parietal layer)

Pericardial space

Myocardium

Endocardium

Trabeculae

INSIDE OF HEART

Line of attachment of fibrous pericardium and reflection of serous pericardium

Fibrous pericardium

Serous pericardium:
Visceral
Parietal

Pericardial space

Diaphragm

S
R — L
I

Fibrous pericardium fused with diaphragm at central tendon

Fibrous pericardium loosely attached to diaphragm

This section of the heart wall shows the fibrous pericardium, the parietal and visceral layers of the serous pericardium (with the pericardial space between them), the myocardium, and the endocardium. Notice that there is fatty connective tissue between the visceral layer of the serous pericardium (epicardium) and the myocardium. Notice also that the endocardium covers beamlike projections of myocardial muscle tissue, called trabeculae.

*I*nterior of the Heart

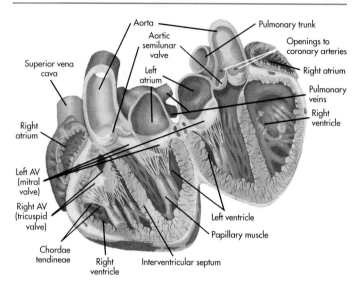

This illustration shows the heart as it would appear if it were cut along a frontal plane and opened like a book. The front portion of the heart lies to the reader's right; the back portion of the heart lies to the reader's left. The four chambers of the heart—two atria and two ventricles—are easily seen.

Chambers and Valves of the Heart

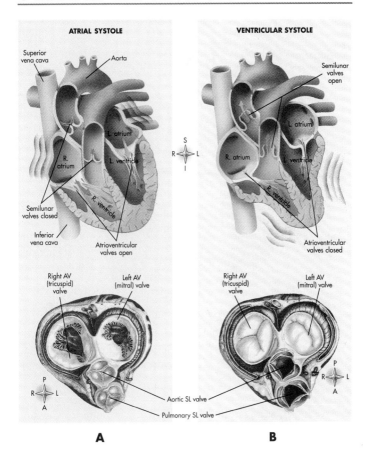

A **B**

The *top illustrations* depict the heart valves as viewed from above. The *bottom illustrations* depict an anterior view cross section of the heart chambers and valves. **A,** The semilunar *(SL)* valves are closed and the atrioventricular *(AV)* valves are open, as when the atria are contracting. **B,** The SL valves are opened and the AV valves are closed, as when the ventricles are contracting.

Coronary Circulation

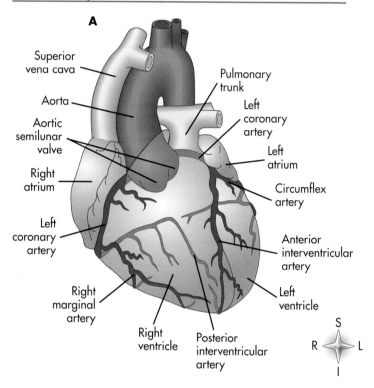

A, Arteries. **B,** Veins. Both illustrations above are anterior views of the heart. Vessels near the anterior surface are more darkly colored than vessels of the posterior surface seen through the heart.

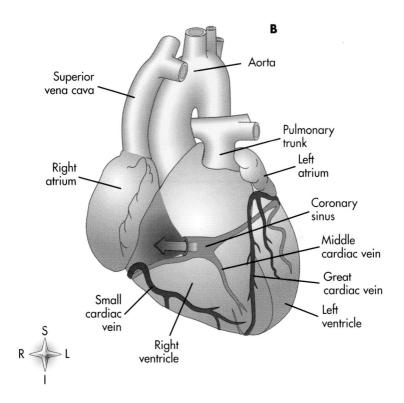

B

Aorta

Superior
vena cava

Pulmonary
trunk

Left
atrium

Right
atrium

Coronary
sinus

Middle
cardiac vein

Great
cardiac vein

Small
cardiac
vein

Left
ventricle

Right
ventricle

S
R ✦ L
I

*S*tructure of Blood Vessels

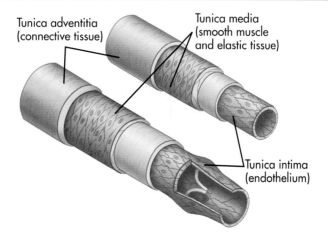

Tunica adventitia
(connective tissue)

Tunica media
(smooth muscle
and elastic tissue)

Tunica intima
(endothelium)

Type of Vessel	Tunica Intima (Endothelium)	Tunica Media (Smooth Muscle; Elastic Connective Tissue)	Tunica Adventitia (Fibrous Connective Tissue)
ARTERIES	Smooth lining	Allows constriction and dilation of vessels; thicker than in veins; muscle innervated by autonomic fibers	Provides flexible support that resists collapse or injury; thicker than in veins; thinner than tunica media
VEINS	Smooth lining with semilunar valves to ensure one-way flow	Allows constriction and dilation of vessels; thinner than in arteries; muscle innervated by autonomic fibers	Provides flexible support that resists collapse or injury; thinner than in arteries; thicker than tunica media
CAPILLARIES	Makes up entire wall of capillary; thinness permits ease of transport across vessel wall	(Absent)	(Absent)

*B*lood Flow Through the Circulatory System

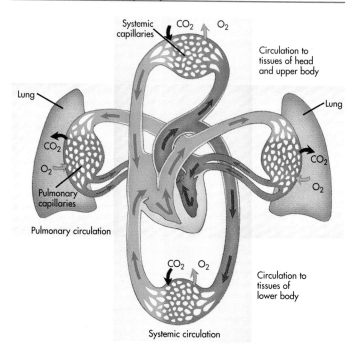

In the pulmonary circulatory route, blood is pumped from the right side of the heart to the gas exchange tissues of the lungs. In the systemic circulation, blood is pumped from the left side of the heart to all other tissues of the body.

Principal Arteries
of the Human Body

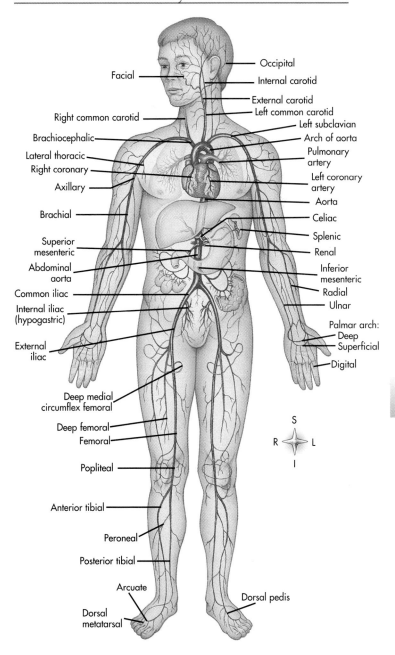

Occipital
Facial
Internal carotid
External carotid
Left common carotid
Right common carotid
Left subclavian
Brachiocephalic
Arch of aorta
Lateral thoracic
Pulmonary artery
Right coronary
Axillary
Left coronary artery
Aorta
Brachial
Celiac
Splenic
Superior mesenteric
Renal
Abdominal aorta
Inferior mesenteric
Common iliac
Radial
Internal iliac (hypogastric)
Ulnar
Palmar arch:
Deep
External iliac
Superficial
Digital
Deep medial circumflex femoral
Deep femoral
Femoral
Popliteal
Anterior tibial
Peroneal
Posterior tibial
Arcuate
Dorsal pedis
Dorsal metatarsal

S
R ✦ L
I

Major Systemic Arteries

Artery*	Region Supplied
ASCENDING AORTA	
Coronary arteries	Myocardium
ARCH OF AORTA	
Brachiocephalic (innominate)	Head and upper extremity
Right subclavian	Head, upper extremity
Right vertebral†	Spinal cord, brain
Right axillary (continuation of subclavian)	Shoulder, chest, axillary region
Right brachial (continuation of axillary)	Arm and hand
Right radial	Lower arm and hand (lateral)
Right ulnar	Lower arm and hand (medial)
Superficial and deep palmar arches (formed by anastomosis of branches of radial and ulnar)	Hand and fingers
Digital	Fingers
Right common carotid	Head and neck
Right internal carotid†	Brain, eye, forehead, nose
Right external carotid†	Thyroid, tongue, tonsils, ear, etc.
Left subclavian	Head and upper extremity
Left vertebral†	Spinal cord, brain
Left axillary (continuation of subclavian)	Shoulder, chest, axillary region
Left brachial (continuation of axillary)	Arm and hand
Left radial	Lower arm and hand (lateral)
Left ulnar	Lower arm and hand (medial)
Superficial and deep palmar arches (formed by anastomosis of branches of radial and ulnar)	Hand and fingers
Digital	Fingers
Left common carotid	Head and neck
Left internal carotid†	Brain, eye, forehead, nose
Left external carotid†	Thyroid, tongue, tonsils, ear, etc.

*Branches of each artery are indented below its name.
†See text and/or figures for branches of the artery.

Artery*	Region Supplied
DESCENDING THORACIC AORTA	
Visceral branches	Thoracic viscera
Bronchial	Lungs, bronchi
Esophageal	Esophagus
Parietal branches	Thoracic walls
Intercostal	Lateral thoracic walls (rib cage)
Superior phrenic	Superior surface of diaphragm
DESCENDING ABDOMINAL AORTA	
Visceral branches	Abdominal viscera
Celiac artery (trunk)	Abdominal viscera
Left gastric	Stomach, esophagus
Common hepatic	Liver
Splenic	Spleen, pancreas, stomach
Superior mesenteric	Pancreas, small intestine, colon
Inferior mesenteric	Descending colon, rectum
Suprarenal	Adrenal (suprarenal) gland
Renal	Kidney
Ovarian	Ovary, uterine tube, ureter
Testicular	Testis, ureter
Parietal branches	Walls of abdomen
Inferior phrenic	Inferior surface of diaphragm, adrenal gland
Lumbar	Lumbar vertebrae and muscles of back
Median sacral	Lower vertebrae
Common iliac (formed by terminal branches of aorta)	Pelvis, lower extremity
External iliac	Thigh, leg, foot
Femoral (continuation of external iliac)	Thigh, leg, foot
Popliteal (continuation of femoral)	Leg, foot
Anterior tibial	Leg, foot
Posterior tibial	Leg, foot
Plantar arch (formed by anastomosis of branches of anterior and posterior tibial arteries)	Foot, toes
Digital	Toes

Continued

$\mathscr{M}$ajor Systemic Arteries—cont'd

Artery*	Region Supplied
DESCENDING ABDOMINAL AORTA—cont'd	
Internal iliac	Pelvis
Visceral branches	Pelvic viscera
Middle rectal	Rectum
Vaginal	Vagina, uterus
Uterine	Uterus, vagina, uterine tube, ovary
Parietal branches	Pelvic wall and external regions
Lateral sacral	Sacrum
Superior gluteal	Gluteal muscles
Obturator	Pubic region, hip joint, groin
Internal pudendal	Rectum, external genitals, floor of pelvis
Inferior gluteal	Lower gluteal region, coccyx, upper thigh

*Branches of each artery are indented below its name.
†See text and/or figures for branches of the artery.

The Aorta

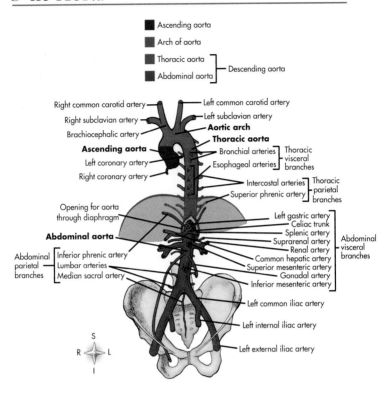

Ascending aorta

Arch of aorta

Thoracic aorta

Abdominal aorta — Descending aorta

Right common carotid artery — — Left common carotid artery
Right subclavian artery — — Left subclavian artery
Brachiocephalic artery — — **Aortic arch**
Ascending aorta — **Thoracic aorta**
Left coronary artery — Bronchial arteries ⎤ Thoracic
Right coronary artery — Esophageal arteries ⎦ visceral branches

Intercostal arteries ⎤ Thoracic
Superior phrenic artery ⎦ parietal branches

Opening for aorta through diaphragm — Left gastric artery
— Celiac trunk
Abdominal aorta — — Splenic artery
— Suprarenal artery ⎤ Abdominal
— Renal artery ⎦ visceral branches
Abdominal ⎡ Inferior phrenic artery — Common hepatic artery
parietal ⎢ Lumbar arteries — Superior mesenteric artery
branches ⎣ Median sacral artery — Gonadal artery
— Inferior mesenteric artery

— Left common iliac artery

— Left internal iliac artery

— Left external iliac artery

S
R ✦ L
I

The aorta is the main systemic artery, serving as a trunk from which other arteries branch. Blood is conducted from the heart first through the ascending aorta, then the arch of the aorta, then through the thoracic and abdominal segments of the descending aorta.

$\mathscr{P}$rincipal Veins of the Human Body

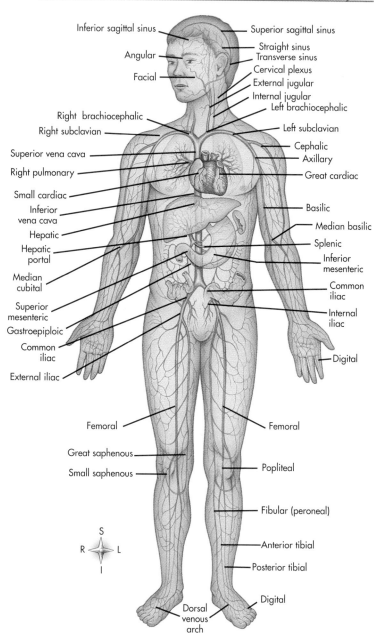

Inferior sagittal sinus

Angular

Facial

Right brachiocephalic

Right subclavian

Superior vena cava

Right pulmonary

Small cardiac

Inferior vena cava

Hepatic

Hepatic portal

Median cubital

Superior mesenteric

Gastroepiploic

Common iliac

External iliac

Superior sagittal sinus

Straight sinus

Transverse sinus

Cervical plexus

External jugular

Internal jugular

Left brachiocephalic

Left subclavian

Cephalic

Axillary

Great cardiac

Basilic

Median basilic

Splenic

Inferior mesenteric

Common iliac

Internal iliac

Digital

Femoral

Great saphenous

Small saphenous

Femoral

Popliteal

Fibular (peroneal)

Anterior tibial

Posterior tibial

Digital

Dorsal venous arch

S

R — L

I

Major Systemic Veins

Vein*	Region Drained
SUPERIOR VENA CAVA	Head, neck, thorax, upper extremity
Brachiocephalic (innominate)	Head, neck, upper extremity
Internal jugular (continuation of sigmoid sinus)	Brain
Lingual	Tongue, mouth
Superior thyroid	Thyroid, deep face
Facial	Superficial face
Sigmoid sinus (continuation of transverse sinus/direct tributary of internal jugular)	Brain, meninges, skull
Superior and inferior petrosal sinuses	Anterior brain, skull
Cavernous sinus	Anterior brain, skull
Ophthalmic veins	Eye, orbit
Transverse sinus (direct tributary of sigmoid sinus)	Brain, meninges, skull
Occipital sinus	Inferior, central region of cranial cavity
Straight sinus	Central region of brain, meninges
Inferior sagittal sinus	Central region of brain, meninges
Superior sagittal (longitudinal) sinus	Superior region of cranial cavity
External jugular	Superficial, posterior head, neck
Subclavian (continuation of axillary/direct tributary of brachiocephalic)	Axilla, lower extremity
Axillary (continuation of basilic/direct tributary of subclavian)	Axilla, lower extremity
Cephalic	Lateral and lower arm, hand
Brachial	Deep arm
Radial	Deep lateral forearm
Ulnar	Deep medial forearm
Basilic (direct tributary of axillary)	Medial and lower arm, hand
Median cubital (basilic) (formed by anastomosis of cephalic and basilic)	Arm, hand

*Tributaries of each vein are indented below its name; deep veins are printed in
dark blue and superficial veins are printed in *light blue*.   *Continued*

*M*ajor Systemic Veins—cont'd

Vein*	Region Drained
SUPERIOR VENA CAVA—cont'd	
Deep and superficial palmar venous arches (formed by anastomosis of cephalic and basilic)	Hand
Digital	Fingers
Azygos (anastomoses with right ascending lumbar)	Right posterior wall of thorax and abdomen, esophagus, bronchi, pericardium, mediastinum
Hemiazygos (anastomoses with left renal)	Left inferior posterior wall of thorax and abdomen, esophagus, mediastinum
Accessory hemiazygos	Left superior posterior wall of thorax
INFERIOR VENA CAVA	Lower trunk and extremity
Phrenic	Diaphragm
Hepatic portal system	Upper abdominal viscera
Hepatic veins (continuations of liver venules and sinusoids and, ultimately, the hepatic portal vein)	Liver
Hepatic portal vein	Gastrointestinal organs, pancreas, spleen, gallbladder
Cystic	Gallbladder
Gastric	Stomach
Splenic	Spleen
Inferior mesenteric	Descending colon, rectum
Pancreatic	Pancreas
Superior mesenteric	Small intestine, most of colon
Gastroepiploic	Stomach
Renal	Kidneys
Suprarenal	Adrenal (suprarenal) gland
Left ovarian	Left ovary
Left testicular	Left testis
Left ascending lumbar (anastomoses with hemiazygos)	Left lumbar region
Right ovarian	Right ovary
Right testicular	Right testis
Right ascending lumbar (anastomoses with azygos)	Right lumbar region

*Tributaries of each vein are indented below its name; deep veins are printed in *dark blue* and superficial veins are printed in *light blue*.

Vein*	Region Drained
INFERIOR VENA CAVA—cont'd	
Common iliac (continuation of external iliac; common iliacs unite to form inferior vena cava)	Lower extremity
External iliac (continuation of femoral/direct tributary of common iliac)	Thigh, leg, foot
Femoral (continuation of popliteal/direct tributary of external iliac)	Thigh, leg, foot
Popliteal	Leg, foot
Posterior tibial	Deep posterior leg
Medial and lateral plantar	Sole of foot
Fibular (peroneal) (continuation of anterior tibial)	Lateral and anterior leg, foot
Anterior tibial	Anterior leg, foot
Dorsal veins of foot	Anterior (dorsal) foot, toes
Small (external, short saphenous	Superficial posterior leg, lateral foot
Great (internal, long) saphenous	Superficial medial and anterior thigh, leg, foot
Dorsal veins of foot	Anterior (dorsal) foot, toes
Dorsal venous arch	Anterior (dorsal) foot, toes
Digital	Toes
Internal iliac	Pelvic region

ℋepatic Portal Circulation

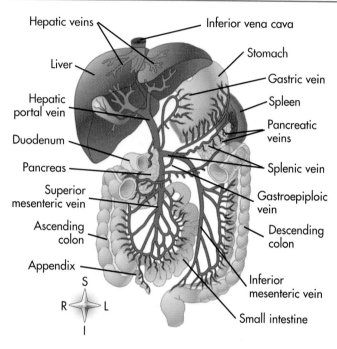

Hepatic veins

Inferior vena cava

Liver

Stomach

Gastric vein

Hepatic portal vein

Spleen

Pancreatic veins

Duodenum

Splenic vein

Pancreas

Superior mesenteric vein

Gastroepiploic vein

Ascending colon

Descending colon

Appendix

Inferior mesenteric vein

Small intestine

S
R—L
I

*M*ajor Veins of the Lower Extremity

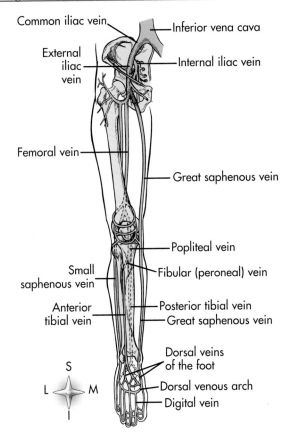

Common iliac vein

Inferior vena cava

External iliac vein

Internal iliac vein

Femoral vein

Great saphenous vein

Popliteal vein

Small saphenous vein

Fibular (peroneal) vein

Anterior tibial vein

Posterior tibial vein

Great saphenous vein

Dorsal veins of the foot

S

L   M

I

Dorsal venous arch

Digital vein

Anterior view of the lower extremity (right leg) showing the major veins.

*F*etal Circulation

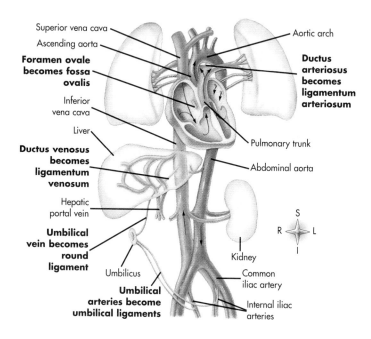

Superior vena cava

Ascending aorta

Foramen ovale becomes fossa ovalis

Inferior vena cava

Liver

Ductus venosus becomes ligamentum venosum

Hepatic portal vein

Umbilical vein becomes round ligament

Umbilicus

Umbilical arteries become umbilical ligaments

Aortic arch

Ductus arteriosus becomes ligamentum arteriosum

Pulmonary trunk

Abdominal aorta

Kidney

Common iliac artery

Internal iliac arteries

S
R ✦ L
I

Before birth, the human circulatory system has several special features that adapt the body to life in the womb. These features *(labeled in bold type)* include two umbilical arteries, one umbilical vein, ductus venosus, foramen ovale, and ductus arteriosus. The placenta, not shown in this illustration, is another essential feature of the fetal circulatory plan.

Conduction System of the Heart

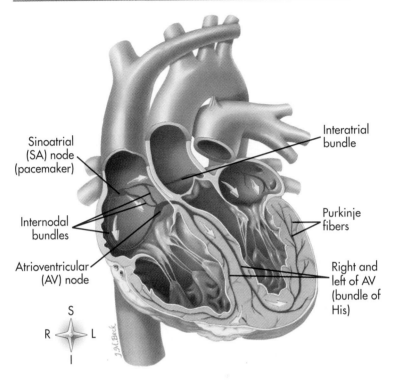

Sinoatrial (SA) node (pacemaker)

Interatrial bundle

Internodal bundles

Purkinje fibers

Atrioventricular (AV) node

Right and left of AV (bundle of His)

Specialized cardiac muscle cells in the wall of the heart rapidly initiate or conduct an electrical impulse throughout the myocardium. The signal is initiated by the sinoatrial (SA) node (pacemaker) and spreads to the rest of right atrial myocardium directly, to the left atrial myocardium by way of a bundle of interatrial conducting fibers, and to the atrioventricular (AV) node by way of three internodal bundles. The AV node then initiates a signal that is conducted through the ventricular myocardium by way of the AV (bundle of His) and Purkinje fibers.

*E*lectrocardiogram

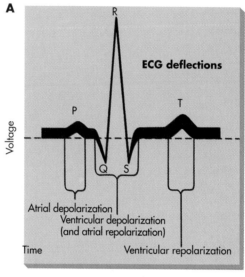

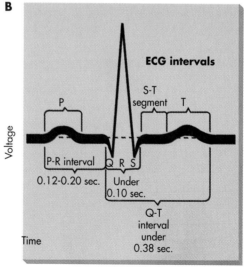

A, An idealized electrocardiogram (ECG) deflection represents depolarization and repolarization of cardiac muscle tissue. **B,** The principal ECG intervals are between P, QRS, and T waves. Note that the P-R interval is measured from the start of the P wave to the start of the Q wave.

Composite Chart of Heart Function

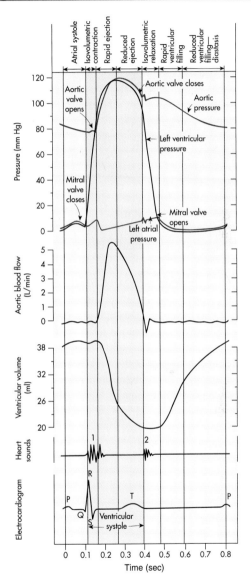

The chart above is a composite of several diagrams of heart function (cardiac pumping cycle, blood pressure, blood flow, volume, heart sounds, and ECG), all adjusted to the same time scale. (From Berne/Levy: *Cardiovascular physiology.*)

Primary Principle of Circulation

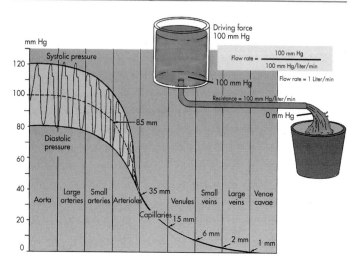

Fluid always travels from an area of high pressure to an area of low pressure. Water flows from an area of high pressure in the tank (100 mm Hg) toward the area of low pressure above the bucket (0 mm Hg). Blood tends to move from an area of high average pressure at the beginning of the aorta (100 mm Hg) toward the area of lowest pressure at the end of the venae cavae (0 mm Hg). Blood flow between any two points in the circulatory system can always be predicted by the pressure gradient.

$\mathcal{R}$elative Blood Volumes

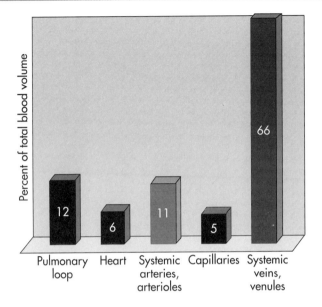

The relative volumes of blood at rest in different parts of the adult cardiovascular system expressed as percentages of total blood volume. Notice that at rest most of the body's blood supply is in the systemic veins and venules.

*V*asomotor Pressoreflexes

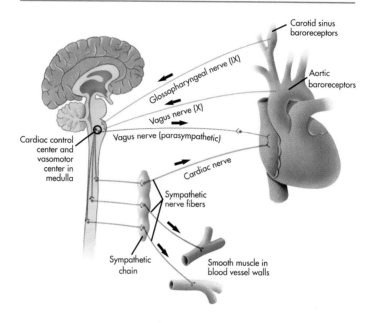

Carotid sinus and aortic baroreceptors detect changes in blood pressure and feed the information back to the cardiac control center and the vasomotor center in the medulla. In response, these control centers alter the ratio between sympathetic and parasympathetic output. If the pressure is too high, a dominance of parasympathetic impulses will reduce it by slowing heart rate, reducing stroke volume, and dilating blood "reservoir" vessels. If the pressure is too low, a dominance of sympathetic impulses will increase it by increasing heart rate and stroke volume and constricting reservoir vessels.

$\mathcal{V}$asomotor Chemoreflexes

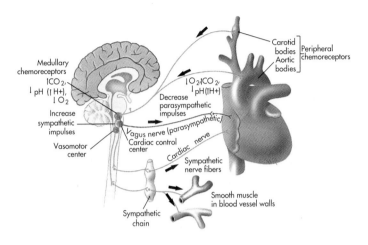

Chemoreceptors in the carotid and aortic bodies, as well as chemoreceptive neurons in the vasomotor center of the medulla itself, detect increases in carbon dioxide (CO_2), decreases in blood oxygen (O_2), and decreases in pH (which is really an increase in H^+). This information feeds back to the cardiac control center and the vasomotor control center of the medulla, which, in turn, alter the ratio of parasympathetic and sympathetic output. When O_2 drops, CO_2 increases, and/or pH drops, a dominance of sympathetic impulses increases heart rate and stroke volume and constricts reservoir vessels, in response.

*S*tarling's Law of the Capillaries

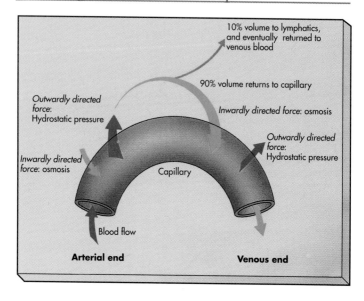

At the arterial end of a capillary the outward driving force of blood pressure is larger than the inwardly directed force of osmosis—thus fluid moves out of the vessel. At the venous end of a capillary the inward driving force of osmosis is greater than the outwardly directed force of hydrostatic pressure—thus fluid enters the vessel. About 90% of the fluid leaving the capillary at the arterial end is recovered by the blood before it leaves the venous end. The remaining 10% is recovered by the venous blood, eventually, by way of the lymphatic vessels.

Mechanisms That Influence Total Plasma Volume

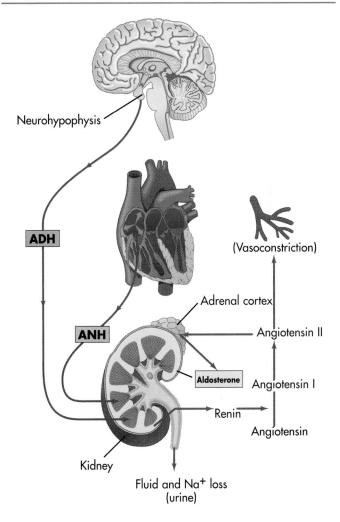

The antidiuretic hormone (ADH) mechanism (1) and renin-angiotensin and aldosterone mechanism (2) tend to increase water retention and thus increase total plasma volume. The atrial natriuretic hormone (ANH) mechanism (3) antagonizes these mechanisms by promoting water loss and thus promoting a decrease in total plasma volume.

Factors That Influence the Flow of Blood

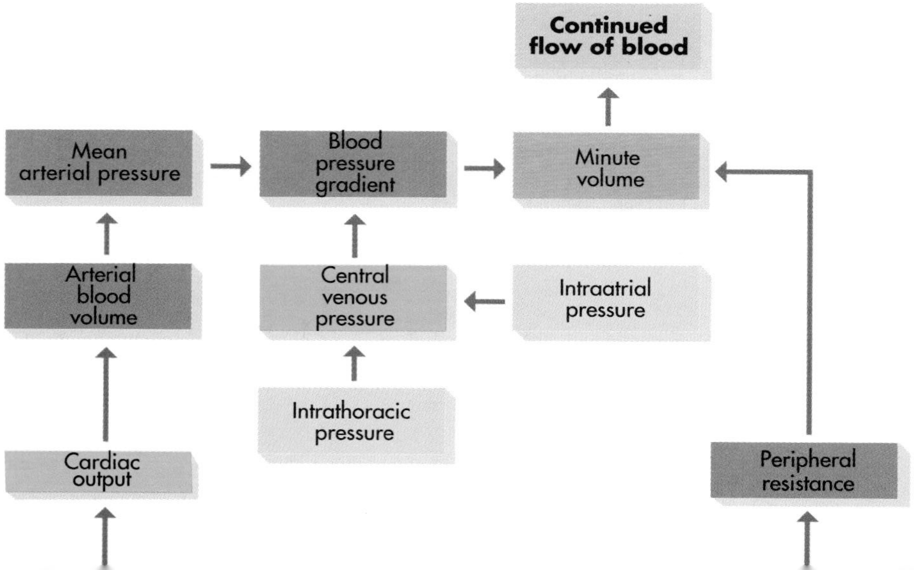

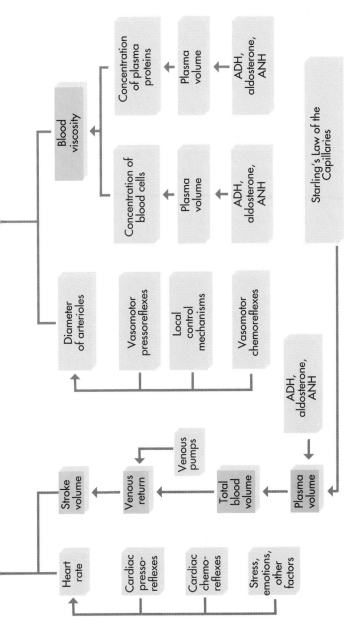

The flow of blood, expressed as volume of blood flowing per minute (or *minute volume*), is determined by various factors. The chart above shows only some of the major factors that influence blood flow. Note that some factors appear more than once in the chart, indicating that they can influence blood flow in several ways.

*P*ulse Points

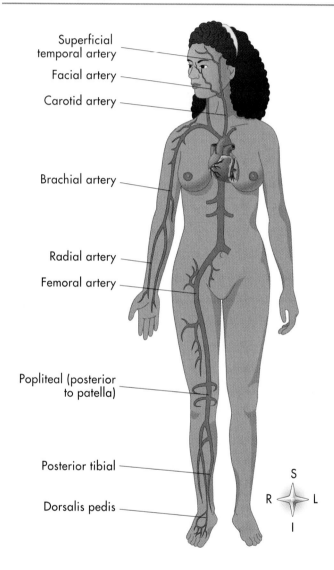

Superficial temporal artery

Facial artery

Carotid artery

Brachial artery

Radial artery

Femoral artery

Popliteal (posterior to patella)

Posterior tibial

Dorsalis pedis

S
R — L
I

Each pulse point is named after the artery with which it is associated.

Lymphatic and Immune System

The two most important functions of the lymphatic system are (1) maintenance of fluid balance in the internal environment and (2) immunity, protection of the body against both external and internal "enemies," such as bacteria and abnormal cell growth. The lymphatic system is actually a specialized component of the circulatory system, since it consists of a moving fluid (lymph) derived from the blood and tissue fluid and a group of vessels (lymphatics) that return the lymph to the blood.

$\mathscr{P}$rincipal Organs of the Lymphatic System

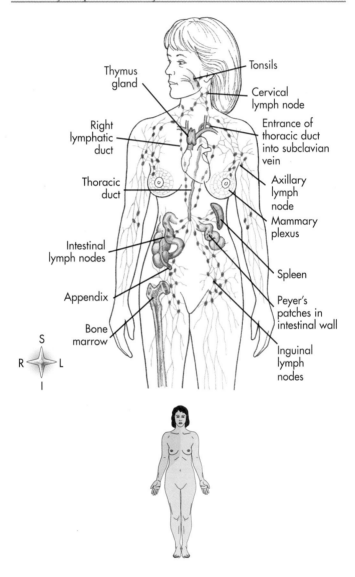

The smaller silhouette shows the areas drained by the right lymphatic duct (*green*) and the thoracic duct (*blue*).

Structure of a Lymph Node

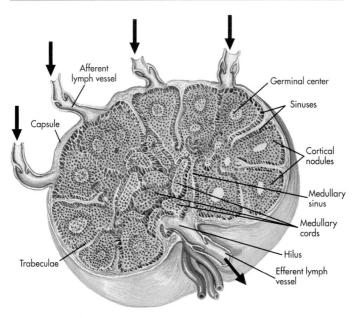

Several afferent valved lymphatics bring lymph to the node. A single efferent lymphatic leaves the node at the hilus. Note that the artery and vein also enter and leave at the hilus. *Arrows* show direction of lymph.

*L*ymphatic Drainage of the Breast

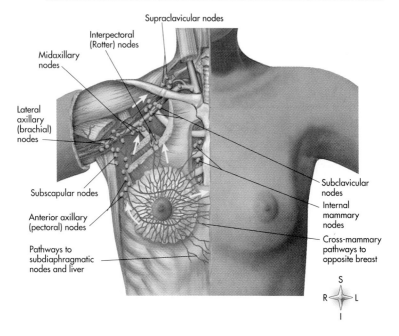

Note the extensive network of lymphatic vessels and nodes that receive lymph from the breast. (From Seidel et al: *Mosby's guide to physical examination*, ed. 4.)

*L*ocation of the Tonsils

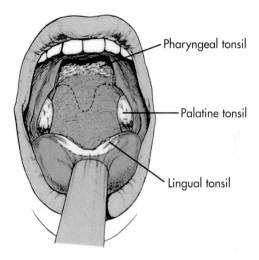

Pharyngeal tonsil

Palatine tonsil

Lingual tonsil

Small segments of the roof and floor of the mouth have been removed to show the protective ring (lymphoid tissue) around the internal openings of the nose and throat.

*T*hymus

The thymus is a primary organ of the lymphatic system. It is an unpaired organ consisting of two pyramidal-shaped lobes with delicate and finely lobulated surfaces.

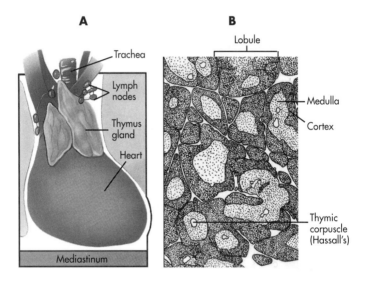

A, Location of the thymus within the mediastinum. **B,** Microscopic structure of the thymus showing several lobules, each with a cortex and a medulla.

Spleen

The spleen has many functions, including defense, hematopoiesis, and red blood cell and platelet destruction; it also serves as a reservoir for blood.

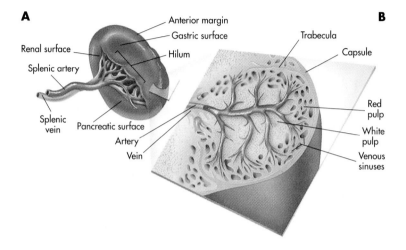

A

Anterior margin
Gastric surface
Hilum
Renal surface
Splenic artery
Splenic vein
Pancreatic surface
Artery
Vein

B

Trabecula
Capsule
Red pulp
White pulp
Venous sinuses

A, Medial aspect of the spleen. Notice the concave surface that fits against the stomach within the abdominopelvic cavity. **B,** Section showing the internal organization of the spleen.

*M*echanisms of Nonspecific Defense

Mechanism	Description
SPECIES RESISTANCE	Genetic characteristics of the human species protect the body from certain pathogens
MECHANICAL AND CHEMICAL BARRIERS	Physical impediments to the entry of foreign cells or substances
Skin and mucosa	Forms a continuous wall that separates the internal environment from the external environment, preventing the entry of pathogens
Secretions	Secretions such as sebum, mucus, and enzymes chemically inhibit the activity of pathogens
INFLAMMATION	The inflammatory response isolates the pathogens and stimulates the speedy arrival of large numbers of immune cells
PHAGOCYTOSIS	Ingestion and destruction of pathogens by phagocytic cells
Neutrophils	Granular leukocytes that are usually the first phagocytic cell to arrive at the scene of an inflammatory response
Macrophages	Monocytes that have enlarged to become giant phagocytic cells capable of consuming many pathogens; often called by other, more specific names when found in specific tissues of the body
NATURAL KILLER (NK) CELLS	Group of lymphocytes that kill many different types of cancer cells and virus-infected cells
INTERFERON	Protein produced by cells after they become infected by a virus; inhibits the spread or further development of a viral infection
COMPLEMENT	Group of plasma proteins (inactive enzymes) that produce a cascade of chemical reactions that ultimately causes lysis (rupture) of a foreign cell; the complement cascade can be triggered by specific or nonspecific immune mechanisms

ℒines of Defense

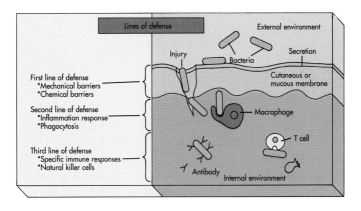

Immune function, that is, defense of the internal environment against foreign cells, proteins, and viruses, includes three layers of protection. The first line of defense is a set of barriers between the internal and external environment, the second line of defense involves the nonspecific inflammatory response (including phagocytosis), and the third line of defense includes the specific immune responses and the nonspecific defense offered by natural killer (NK) cells. Of course, tumor cells that arise in the body are already past the first two lines of defense and must be attacked by the third line of defense. The diagram above is a simplification of the complex function of the immune system; in reality, there is a great deal of crossover of mechanisms between these "lines of defense."

*In*flammatory Response

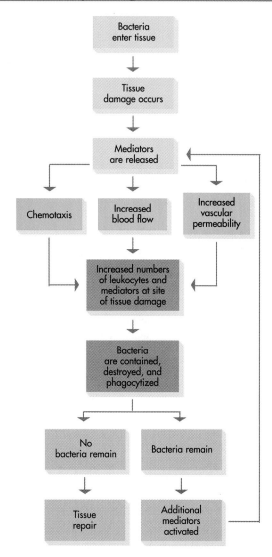

Tissue damage caused by bacteria triggers a series of events that produces the inflammatory response and promotes phagocytosis at the site of injury. These responses tend to inhibit or destroy the bacteria.

$\mathscr{B}$-Cell Development

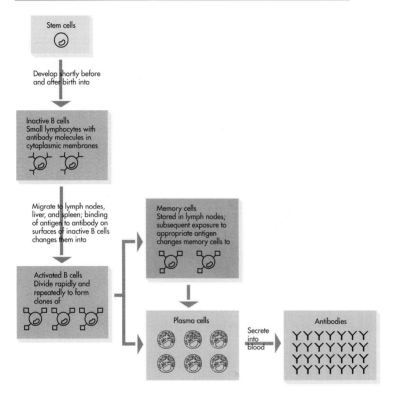

B-cell development takes place in two stages. *First stage:* shortly before and after birth, stem cells develop into inactive B cells. *Second stage* (occurs only if inactive B cell contacts its specific antigen): inactive B cell develops into activated B cell, which divides rapidly and repeatedly to form a clone of plasma cells and a clone of memory cells. Plasma cells secrete antibodies capable of combining with specific antigens that cause inactive B cells to develop into active B cells. Stem cells maintain a constant population of newly differentiating cells.

*S*tructure of the Antibody Molecule

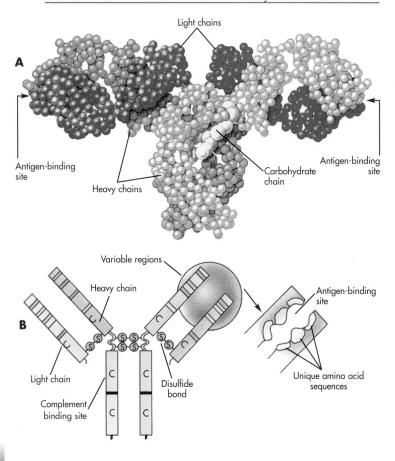

A, In this molecular model of a typical antibody molecule, the light chains are represented by strands of *red spheres* (each represents an individual amino acid). Heavy chains are represented by strands of *blue spheres.* Notice that the heavy chains can complex with a carbohydrate chain. **B,** This simplified diagram shows the variable regions, highlighted by *colored bars,* that represent amino acid sequences unique to that molecule. Constant regions of the heavy and light chains are marked "*C.*" The *inset* at the right shows that the variable regions at the end of each arm of the molecule form a cleft that serves as an antigen–binding site.

Actions of Antibodies

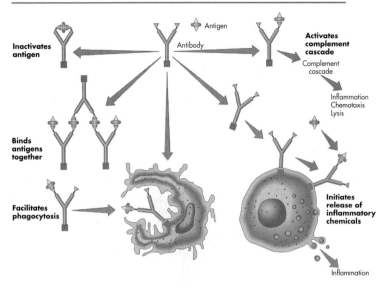

Antibodies act on antigens by inactivating and bending them together to facilitate phagocytosis and by initiating inflammation and activating the complement cascade.

*C*omplement Fixation

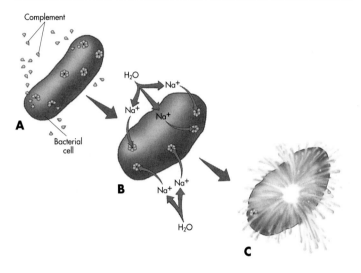

A, Complement molecules activated by antibodies form doughnut-shaped complexes in a bacterium's plasma membrane. **B,** Holes in the complement complex allow sodium (Na^+) and then water (H_2O) to diffuse into the bacterium. **C,** After enough water has entered, the swollen bacterium bursts.

$\mathcal{T}$-Cell Development

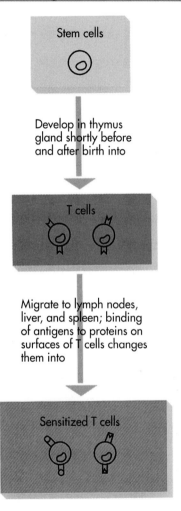

The *first stage* of T-cell development occurs in the thymus gland shortly before and after birth. Stem cells maintain a constant population of newly differentiating cells as they are needed. The *second stage* occurs only if a T cell is presented an antigen, which combines with certain proteins on the T cell's surface.

$\mathscr{S}$timulation and Effects of T Cells

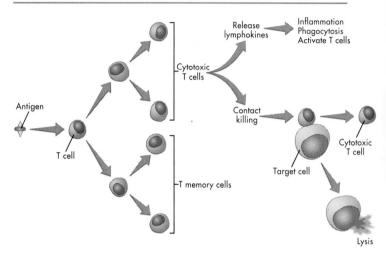

When presented with an antigen, stimulated T cells form either cytotoxic T or memory T cells that cause contact killing or release of lymphokines or produce antibody-producing T memory cells.

$\mathcal{T}$ Cell Function

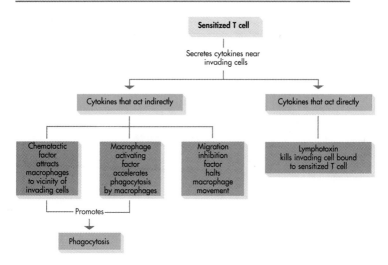

Sensitized T cells produce cell-mediated immunity by releasing various compounds in the vicinity of invading cells. Some act directly and some act indirectly to kill invading cells.

*C*ytotoxic T Cells

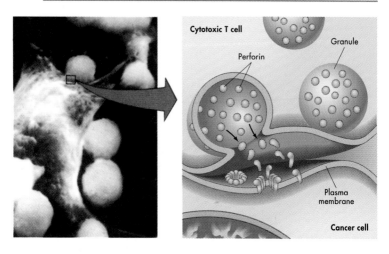

The *blue spheres* seen in this scanning electron microscope view are cytotoxic T cells attacking a much larger cancer cell. T cells are a significant part of the human body's defense against cancer and other abnormal or foreign cells. The *inset* shows how the lymphotoxin *perforin* acts to kill cells by puncturing holes in their plasma membranes.

Types of Specific Immunity

Type	Description or Example
INHERITED IMMUNITY	Immunity to certain diseases develops before birth; also called inborn immunity
ACQUIRED IMMUNITY	
Natural immunity	Exposure to the causative agent is not deliberate
Active (exposure)	A child develops measles and acquires an immunity to a subsequent infection
Passive (exposure)	A fetus receives protection from the mother through the placenta, or an infant receives protection via the mother's milk
Artificial immunity	Exposure to the causative agent is deliberate
Active (exposure)	Injection of the causative agent, such as a vaccination against polio, confers immunity
Passive (exposure)	Injection of protective material (antibodies) that was developed by another individual's immune system

12

Respiratory
System

The respiratory system functions as an air distributor and a gas exchanger so that oxygen may be supplied to and carbon dioxide removed from the body's cells.

Structural Plan of the Respiratory System

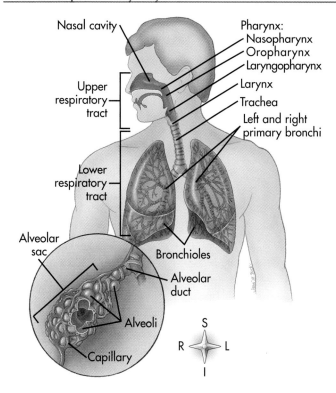

The *inset* in the illustration above shows the alveolar sacs where the interchange of oxygen and carbon dioxide takes place through the walls of the grapelike alveoli. Capillaries surround the alveoli.

Pharynx

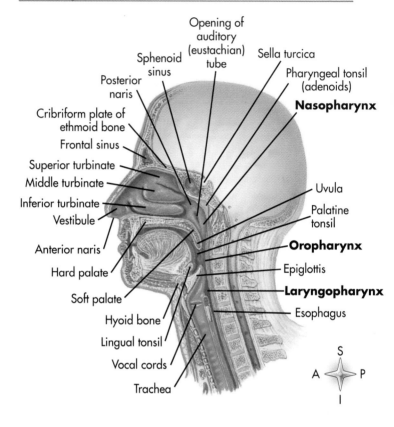

Opening of
auditory
(eustachian)
tube

Sphenoid
sinus

Posterior
naris

Cribriform plate of
ethmoid bone

Frontal sinus

Superior turbinate

Middle turbinate

Inferior turbinate

Vestibule

Anterior naris

Hard palate

Soft palate

Hyoid bone

Lingual tonsil

Vocal cords

Trachea

Sella turcica

Pharyngeal tonsil
(adenoids)

Nasopharynx

Uvula

Palatine
tonsil

Oropharynx

Epiglottis

Laryngopharynx

Esophagus

S
A P
I

This midsagittal section shows the three divisions of the pharynx (nasopharynx, oropharynx, and laryngopharynx) and nearby
structures.

Anatomy of the Larynx

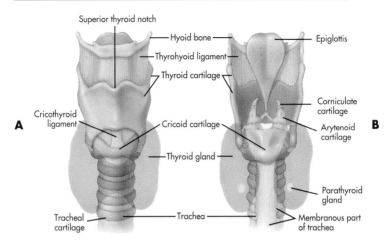

Superior thyroid notch

Hyoid bone

Thyrohyoid ligament

Thyroid cartilage

Epiglottis

Corniculate cartilage

Cricothyroid ligament

Cricoid cartilage

Arytenoid cartilage

Thyroid gland

Parathyroid gland

Tracheal cartilage

Trachea

Membranous part of trachea

A

B

A, Anterior view of the larynx. **B,** Posterior view of the larynx.

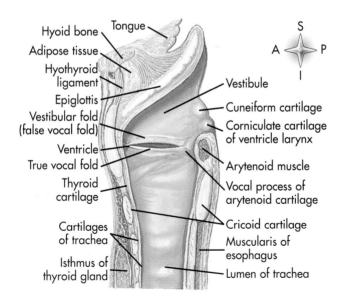

Hyoid bone

Tongue

Adipose tissue

Hyothyroid ligament

Epiglottis

Vestibular fold (false vocal fold)

Ventricle

True vocal fold

Thyroid cartilage

Cartilages of trachea

Isthmus of thyroid gland

Vestibule

Cuneiform cartilage

Corniculate cartilage of ventricle larynx

Arytenoid muscle

Vocal process of arytenoid cartilage

Cricoid cartilage

Muscularis of esophagus

Lumen of trachea

S A P I

Sagittal section of the larynx.

*V*ocal Cords

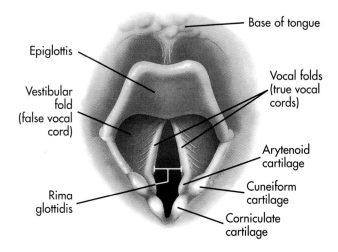

This illustrates an endoscopic view of the vocal cords and related structures, as viewed from above.

$\mathcal{L}$obes and Segments of the Lungs

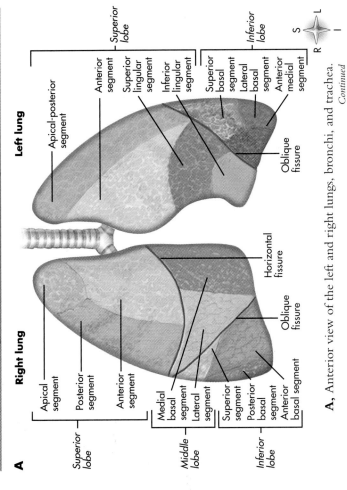

Right lung

Superior lobe
- Apical segment
- Posterior segment
- Anterior segment

Middle lobe
- Medial basal segment
- Lateral segment

Inferior lobe
- Superior segment
- Posterior basal segment
- Anterior basal segment

Horizontal fissure

Oblique fissure

Left lung

Superior lobe
- Apical-posterior segment
- Anterior segment
- Superior lingular segment
- Inferior lingular segment

Inferior lobe
- Superior basal segment
- Lateral basal segment
- Anterior medial segment

Oblique fissure

A, Anterior view of the left and right lungs, bronchi, and trachea.
Continued

S
R — L
I

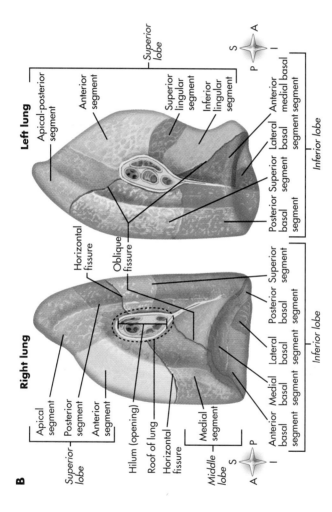

B, Medial views of the right and left lungs.

The Gas-Exchange Structures of the Lung

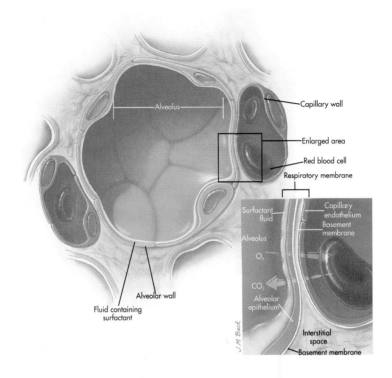

Each alveolus is continually ventilated with fresh air. The *inset* in the illustration above shows a magnified view of the respiratory membrane composed of the alveolar wall (fluid coating, epithelial cells, and basement membrane), interstitial fluid, and the wall of a pulmonary capillary (basement membrane and endothelial cells). The gases, CO_2 (carbon dioxide) and O_2 (oxygen), diffuse across the respiratory membrane.

*M*echanics of Ventilation

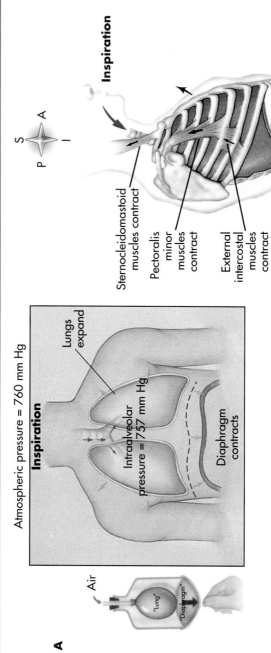

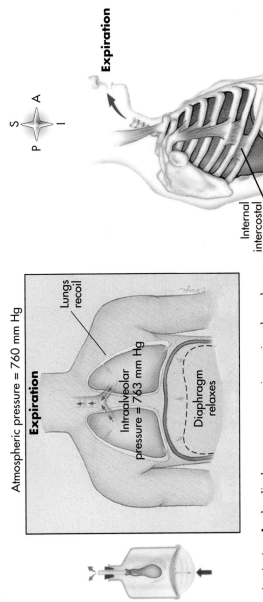

Atmospheric pressure = 760 mm Hg

Expiration

Lungs recoil

Intraalveolar pressure = 763 mm Hg

Diaphragm relaxes

B

Expiration

S · A · P · I

Internal intercostal muscles contract

Diaphragm relaxes

Abdominal muscles contract

During *inspiration,* **A,** the diaphragm contracts, increasing the volume of the thoracic cavity. This increase in volume results in a decrease in pressure, which causes air to rush into the lungs. During *expiration,* **B,** the diaphragm returns to an upward position, reducing the volume in the thoracic cavity. Air pressure increases then, forcing air out of the lungs. *Insets* show the classic model in which a jar represents the rib cage, a rubber sheet represents the diaphragm, and a balloon represents the lungs.

*P*ulmonary Volumes and Capacities

The volumes of air moved in and out of the lungs and remaining in them must be normal so that a normal exchange of oxygen and carbon dioxide can occur between alveolar air and pulmonary capillary blood.

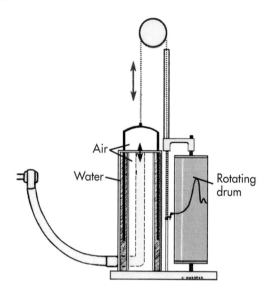

Spirometers are devices that measure the volume of gas that the lungs inhale and exhale, usually as a function of time. The diagram above of a classic spirometer design shows how the volume of air exhaled and inhaled is recorded as a rising and falling line.

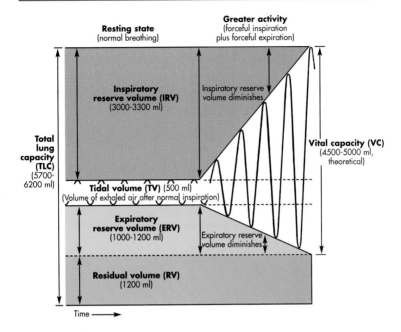

A spirogram is a graphic recording of the changing pulmonary volumes observed during breathing. During normal, quiet respirations the atmosphere and lungs exchange about 500 ml of air (TV). With a forcible inspiration, about 3,300 ml more air can be inhaled (IRV). After a normal inspiration and normal expiration, approximately 1,000 ml more air can be forcibly expired (ERV). Vital capacity is the amount of air that can be forcibly expired after a maximal inspiration and indicates, therefore, the largest amount of air that can enter and leave the lungs during respiration. Residual volume is the air that remains trapped in the alveoli.

Pulmonary Volumes and Capacities—cont'd

Volume	Description	Typical Value	Capacity	Formula	Typical Value
Tidal volume (TV)	Volume moved into or out of the respiratory tract during a normal respiratory cycle	500 ml	Vital capacity (VC)	TV + IRV + ERV	4,500–5,000 ml
Inspiratory reserve volume (IRV)	Maximum volume that can be moved into the respiratory tract after a normal inspiration	3,000–3,300 ml	Inspiratory capacity (IC)	TV + IRV	3,500–3,800 ml
Expiratory reserve volume (ERV)	Maximum volume that can be moved out of the respiratory tract after a normal expiration	1,000–1,200 ml	Functional residual capacity (FRC)	ERV + RV	2,200–2,400 ml
Residual volume (RV)	Volume remaining in the respiratory tract after maximum expiration	1,200 ml	Total lung capacity (TLC)	TV + IRV + ERV + RV	5,700–6,200 ml

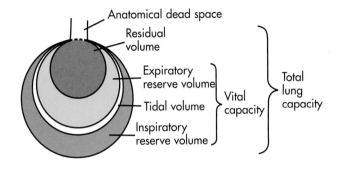

This figure shows the pulmonary volumes at rest as relative proportions of an inflated balloon.

$\mathcal{O}$xygen and Carbon Dioxide Pressure Gradients

	Atmosphere	Alveolar Air	Systemic Arterial Blood	Systemic Venous Blood
P_{O_2}	160*	100	100	40
P_{CO_2}	0.2	40	40	46

*Figures indicate approximate mm Hg pressure under usual conditions.

Hemoglobin

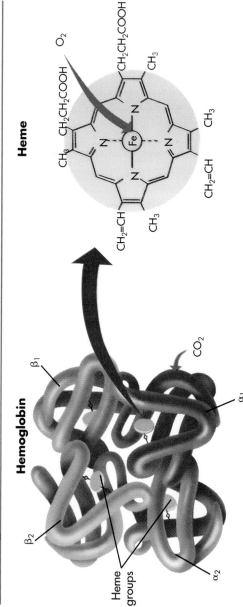

Hemoglobin is a quaternary protein, consisting of four different tertiary (folded) polypeptide chains—two alpha (α) chains and two beta (β) chains. Each chain has an associated iron-containing heme group, as seen in detail in the *inset*. Oxygen (O_2) can bind to the iron (Fe) of the heme group, or carbon dioxide (CO_2) can bind to amine groups of the amino acids in the polypeptide chains.

$\mathscr{O}$xygen–Hemoglobin Dissociation Curve

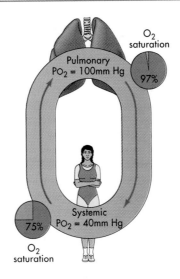

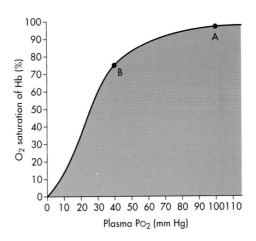

The *graph* above represents the relationship between PO_2 and O_2 saturation of hemoglobin (Hb-O_2 affinity). The *inset* shows how the graphed curve relates to oxygen transport by the blood. Notice that at high plasma PO_2 values (*point A*), hemoglobin (Hb) is fully loaded with oxygen. At low plasma PO_2 values (*point B*), Hb is only partially loaded with oxygen.

Carbon Dioxide-Hemoglobin Reaction

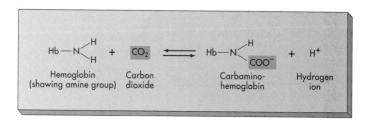

Hemoglobin (showing amine group) + Carbon dioxide ⇌ Carbamino-hemoglobin + Hydrogen ion

Carbon dioxide can bind to an amine group (NH_2) in an amino acid within a hemoglobin (Hb) molecule to form carbaminohemoglobin ($HbNCOOH^-$) and a hydrogen ion. The *highlighted areas* show where the original carbon dioxide molecule is in each part of the equation.

Carbon Dioxide Dissociation Curve

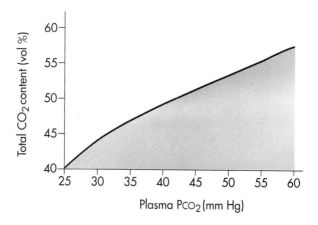

The relationship between PCO_2 and total CO_2 content (vol %) is graphed as a nearly straight line. Notice that the CO_2-carrying capacity of blood increases as the plasma PCO_2 increases.

$\mathcal{F}$ormation of Bicarbonate

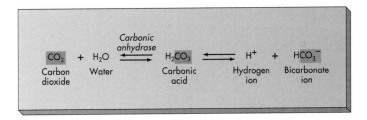

Carbon dioxide can react with water to form carbonic acid, a reaction catalyzed by the red blood cell (RBC) enzyme *carbonic anhydrase*. Carbonic acid then dissociates to form bicarbonate and a hydrogen ion. The *highlighted areas* show where the original carbon dioxide molecule is in each part of the equation. The *double arrows* show that each reaction is reversible, the actual rate in each direction governed by the relative concentration of each molecule.

Carbon Dioxide Transport in the Blood

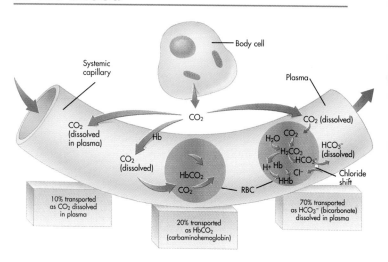

As the illustration above shows, CO_2 dissolves in the plasma. Some of the dissolved CO_2 enters RBCs and combines with Hb to form carbaminohemoglobin ($HbCO_2$). Some of the CO_2 entering RBCs combines with H_2O to form carbonic acid (H_2CO_3), a process facilitated by an enzyme (carbonic anhydrase) present inside each cell. Carbonic acid then dissociates to form H^+ and bicarbonate (HCO_3^-). The H^+ combines with Hb, while the HCO_3^- diffuses down its concentration gradient into the plasma. As HCO_3^- leaves each RBC, Cl^- enters and prevents an imbalance in charge—a phenomenon called the chloride shift.

Blood Oxygen

	Systemic Venous Blood	Systemic Arterial Blood
Po_2	40 mm Hg	100 mm Hg
Oxygen saturation	75%	97%
Oxygen content	15 ml O_2 per 100 ml blood	20 ml O_2 per 100 ml blood*

*Oxygen use by tissues = Difference between oxygen contents of arterial and venous blood (20-15) = 5 ml O_2 per 100 ml blood circulated per minute.

$\mathcal{O}$xygen Dissociation Curve for Oxygen-Binding Proteins

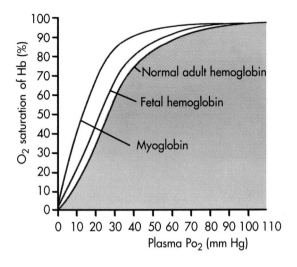

Both fetal hemoglobin and myoglobin have oxygen dissociation curves that are shifted to the left of the curve for normal adult hemoglobin. Thus both of the molecules attract and hold oxygen more strongly than normal adult hemoglobin.

*I*nteraction of P_{O_2} and P_{CO_2} on Gas Transport by the Blood

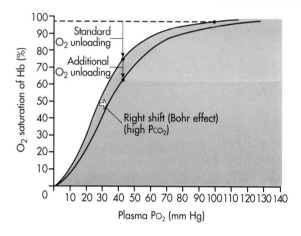

The increased P_{CO_2} in systemic tissues decreases the affinity between Hb and O_2, shown as a right shift of the oxygen-hemoglobin dissociation curve. This phenomenon is known as the *Bohr effect*. A right shift can also be caused by a decrease in plasma pH.

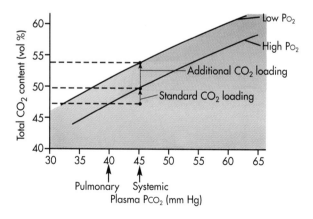

The decreased P_{O_2} commonly observed in systemic tissues increases the CO_2 content of the blood, shown here as a left shift of the CO_2 dissociation curve. This phenomenon is known as the *Haldane effect*.

$\mathscr{S}$cheme of Respiratory Regulation

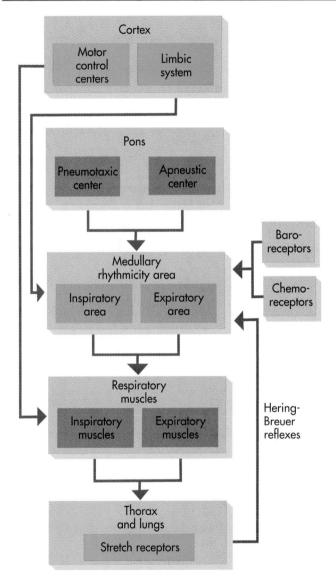

The diagram above summarizes the fact that the actions of the respiratory muscles are governed by control centers in the medulla with feedback or other input from other regions of the nervous system.

Digestive System

The process of altering the chemical and physical composition of food so that it can be absorbed and used by the body cells (known as digestion) is the function of the digestive system. The process of digestion depends on both endocrine and exocrine secretions and the controlled movement of ingested food materials through the tract so that absorption can occur.

Organs of the Digestive System

Segments of the Gastrointestinal Tract	Accessory Organs
Mouth	Salivary glands
Oropharynx	Parotid
Esophagus	Submandibular
Stomach	Sublingual
Small intestine	Tongue
Duodenum	Teeth
Jejunum	Liver
Ileum	Gallbladder
Large intestine	Pancreas
Cecum	Vermiform appendix
Colon	
Ascending colon	
Transverse colon	
Descending colon	
Sigmoid colon	
Rectum	
Anal canal	

Location of Digestive Organs in the Body

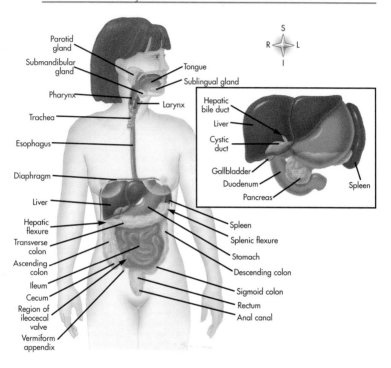

*W*all of the GI Tract

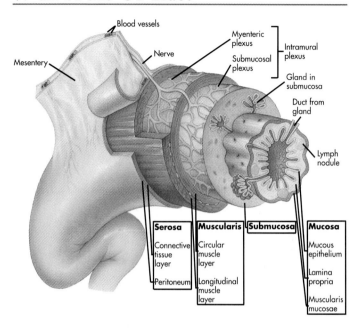

The wall of the gastrointestinal (GI) tract is made up of four layers, shown above in a generalized diagram of a segment of the GI tract. Notice that the serosa is continuous with a fold of serous membrane called a *mesentery*. Notice also that digestive glands may empty their products into the lumen of the GI tract by way of ducts.

Modifications of Layers of the Digestive Tract Wall

Organ	Mucosa	Muscularis	Serosa
Esophagus	Stratified squamous epithelium resists abrasion	Two layers—inner one of circular fibers and outer one of longitudinal fibers; striated muscle in upper part and smooth muscle in lower part of esophagus and in rest of tract	Outer layer fibrous (adventitia); serous around part of esophagus in thoracic cavity
Stomach	Arranged in flexible longitudinal folds, called *rugae*; allow for distention; contains gastric pits with microscopic gastric glands	Has three layers instead of usual two—circular, longitudinal, and oblique fibers; two sphincters—lower esophageal at entrance of stomach and pyloric at its exit, formed by circular fibers	Outer layer, visceral peritoneum; hangs in double fold from lower edge of stomach over intestines, forming apronlike structure; greater omentum; lesser omentum connects stomach to liver
Small intestine	Contains permanent circular folds, plicae circulares Microscopic fingerlike projections, villi with brush border	Two layers—inner one of circular fibers and outer one of longitudinal fibers	Outer layer, visceral peritoneum, continuous with mesentery

Small intestine—cont'd	Crypts (of Lieberkühn) Microscopic duodenal (Brunner's) mucous glands Clusters of lymph nodules (Peyer's patches) Numerous single lymph nodes, called solitary nodes	
Large intestine	Solitary lymph nodes Intestinal mucous glands Anal columns form in anal region	Outer longitudinal layer condensed to form three tapelike strips (taeniae coli); small sacs (haustra) give rest of wall of large intestine puckered appearance; internal anal sphincter formed by circular smooth fibers; external anal sphincter formed by striated fibers	Outer layer, visceral peritoneum, continuous with mesocolon

The Oral Cavity

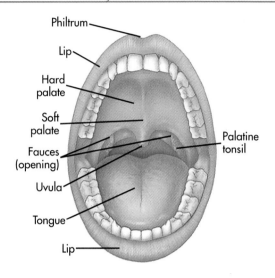

The Tongue

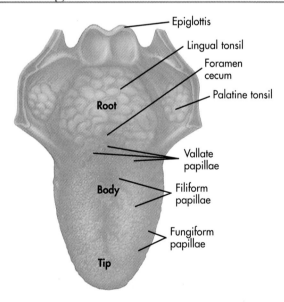

Dorsal surface of the tongue.

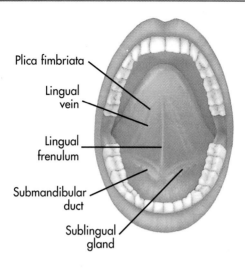

Plica fimbriata

Lingual vein

Lingual frenulum

Submandibular duct

Sublingual gland

The mouth cavity, showing the ventral surface of the tongue.

Salivary Glands

Three pairs of compound tubuloalveolar glands secrete a major amount (about 1 liter) of the saliva produced by the human body each day.

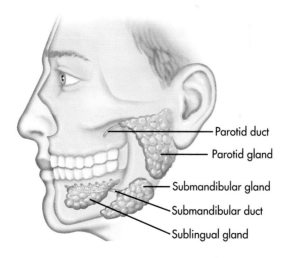

Parotid duct

Parotid gland

Submandibular gland

Submandibular duct

Sublingual gland

Lateral view of the head, showing the location of the salivary glands.

*T*eeth

The teeth are the organs of *mastication,* or chewing.

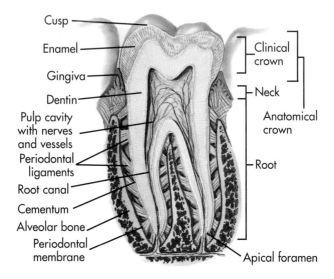

A molar tooth sectioned to show its bony socket and details of its three main parts: crown, neck, and root. Enamel (over the crown) and cementum (over the neck and root) surround the dentin layer. The pulp contains nerves and blood vessels.

*D*entition

| | Number Per Jaw | |
Name of Tooth	Deciduous Set	Permanent Set
Central incisors	2	2
Lateral incisors	2	2
Canines (cuspids)	2	2
Premolars (bicuspids)	0	4
First molars (tricuspids)	2	2
Second molars	2	2
Third molars (wisdom teeth)	0	2
TOTAL (per jaw)	10	16
TOTAL (per set)	20	32

Deciduous teeth

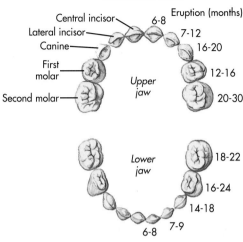

Central incisor — 6-8
Lateral incisor — 7-12
Canine — 16-20
First molar — 12-16
Second molar — 20-30

Eruption (months)

Upper jaw

Lower jaw

18-22
16-24
14-18
6-8   7-9

Adult teeth

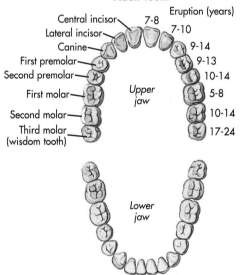

Central incisor — 7-8
Lateral incisor — 7-10
Canine — 9-14
First premolar — 9-13
Second premolar — 10-14
First molar — 5-8
Second molar — 10-14
Third molar (wisdom tooth) — 17-24

Eruption (years)

Upper jaw

Lower jaw

In the deciduous (baby) set of teeth, there are no premolars and only two pairs of molars in each jaw. Generally the lower teeth erupt before the corresponding upper teeth.

*S*tomach

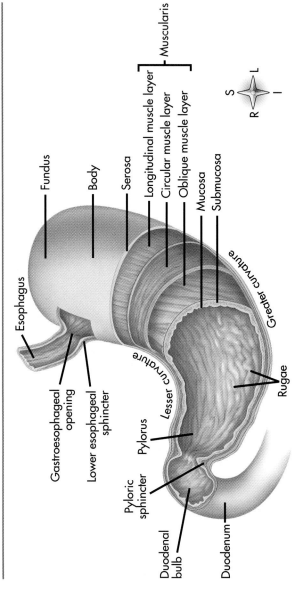

Esophagus

Fundus

Body

Serosa

Muscularis

Longitudinal muscle layer

Circular muscle layer

Oblique muscle layer

Mucosa

Submucosa

Gastroesophageal opening

Lower esophageal sphincter

Lesser curvature

Greater curvature

Pylorus

Pyloric sphincter

Duodenal bulb

Duodenum

Rugae

S

R L

I

Gastric Pits and Gastric Glands

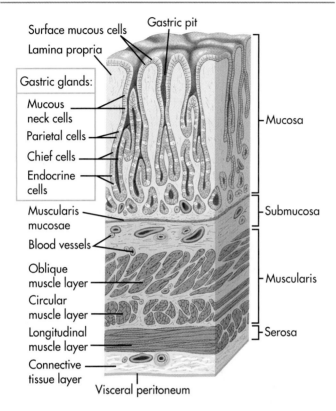

Surface mucous cells

Gastric pit

Lamina propria

Gastric glands:

Mucous neck cells

Parietal cells

Chief cells

Endocrine cells

Muscularis mucosae

Blood vessels

Oblique muscle layer

Circular muscle layer

Longitudinal muscle layer

Connective tissue layer

Visceral peritoneum

Mucosa

Submucosa

Muscularis

Serosa

Gastric pits are depressions in the epithelial lining of the stomach. At the bottom of each pit is one or more tubular *gastric glands.* Chief cells produce the enzymes of gastric juice, and parietal cells produce stomach acid.

Wall of the Small Intestine

Segment of jejunum

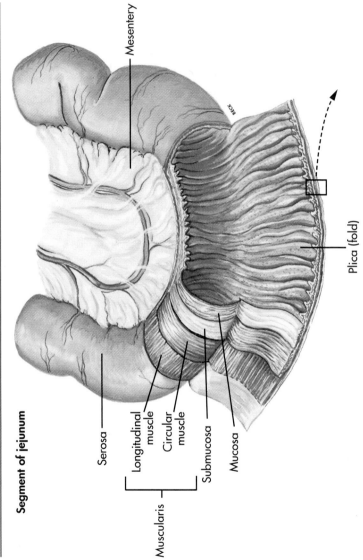

Mesentery

Plica (fold)

Serosa

Longitudinal muscle

Circular muscle

Submucosa

Mucosa

Muscularis

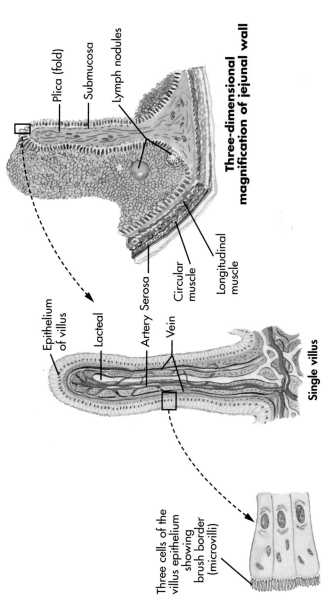

Plica (fold)

Submucosa

Lymph nodules

**Three-dimensional
magnification of jejunal wall**

Circular
muscle

Longitudinal
muscle

Epithelium
of villus

Lacteal

Artery   Serosa

Vein

Single villus

Three cells of the
villus epithelium
showing
brush border
(microvilli)

Note that the folds of mucosa are covered with villi and each villus is covered with epithelium, which increases the surface area for absorption of food.

$\mathscr{D}$ivisions of the Large Intestine

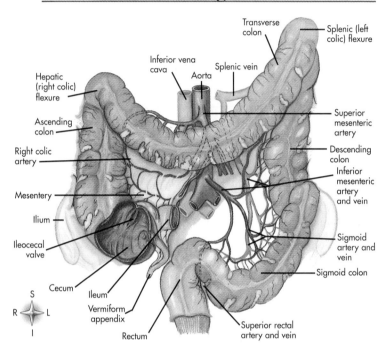

Transverse colon

Splenic (left colic) flexure

Inferior vena cava

Aorta

Splenic vein

Hepatic (right colic) flexure

Ascending colon

Right colic artery

Mesentery

Ilium

Ileocecal valve

Cecum

Ileum

Vermiform appendix

Rectum

Superior mesenteric artery

Descending colon

Inferior mesenteric artery and vein

Sigmoid artery and vein

Sigmoid colon

Superior rectal artery and vein

S
R — L
I

The Rectum and Anus

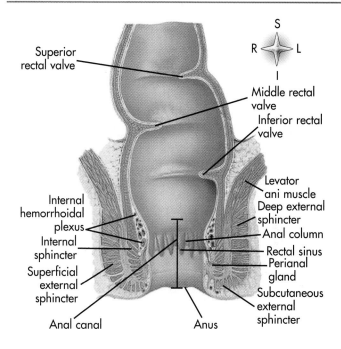

Superior rectal valve

S

R — L

I

Middle rectal valve

Inferior rectal valve

Levator ani muscle

Internal hemorrhoidal plexus

Deep external sphincter

Internal sphincter

Anal column

Rectal sinus

Superficial external sphincter

Perianal gland

Anal canal

Subcutaneous external sphincter

Anus

Peritoneum

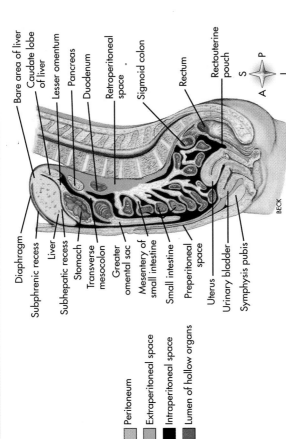

Diaphragm
Subphrenic recess
Liver
Subhepatic recess
Stomach
Transverse mesocolon
Greater omental sac
Mesentery of small intestine
Small intestine
Preperitoneal space
Uterus
Urinary bladder
Symphysis pubis

Bare area of liver
Caudate lobe of liver
Lesser omentum
Pancreas
Duodenum
Retroperitoneal space
Sigmoid colon
Rectum
Rectouterine pouch

BECK

Peritoneum
Extraperitoneal space
Intraperitoneal space
Lumen of hollow organs

This sagittal view of the abdomen shows the peritoneum and its reflections. *Intraperitoneal* spaces are shown in *black* and *extraperitoneal* spaces in *green*. The portion of the extraperitoneal space along the posterior wall of the abdomen is often called the *retroperitoneal space*.

Gross Structure of the Liver

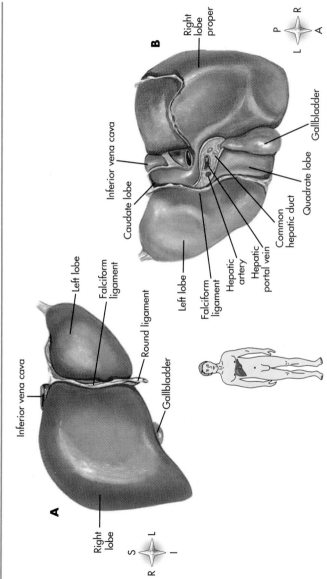

A, Anterior view of the liver. **B,** Inferior view of the liver.

Microscopic Structure of the Liver

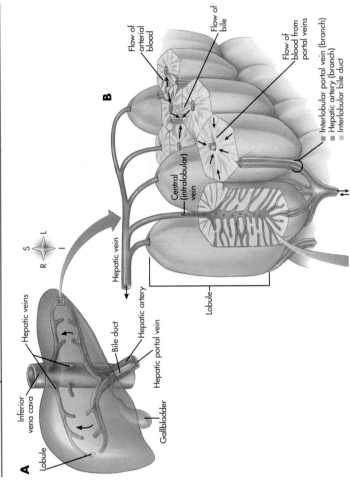

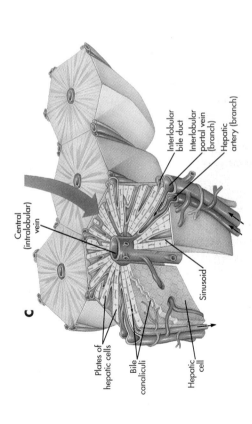

A, This diagram shows the location of the liver lobules relative to the overall circulatory scheme of the liver. **B** and **C,** Enlarged views of several lobules show how blood from the hepatic portal veins and hepatic arteries flows through sinusoids and thus past plates of hepatic cells toward a central vein in each lobule. Hepatic cells form bile, which flows through bile canaliculi toward hepatic ducts that eventually drain the bile from the liver.

Common Bile Duct and its Tributaries

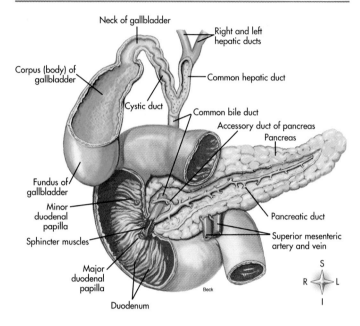

Obstruction of either the hepatic or the common bile duct by stone or spasm prevents bile from being ejected into the duodenum.

*P*ancreas

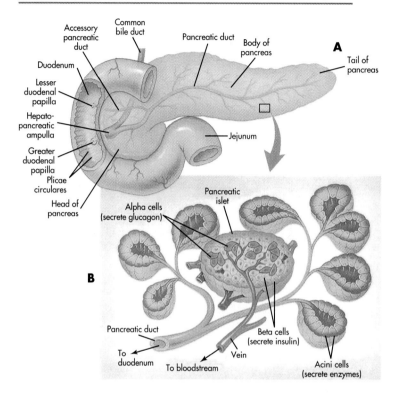

A, Pancreas dissected to show main and accessory ducts. The main duct may join the common bile duct, as shown here, to enter the duodenum by a single opening at the major duodenal papilla, or the two ducts may have separate openings. The accessory pancreatic duct is usually present and has a separate opening into the duodenum. **B,** Exocrine glandular cells (around small pancreatic ducts) and endocrine glandular cells of pancreatic islets (adjacent to blood capillaries). Exocrine pancreatic cells secrete pancreatic juice, alpha endocrine cells secrete glucagon, and beta cells secrete insulin.

*T*ransverse Section of the Abdomen

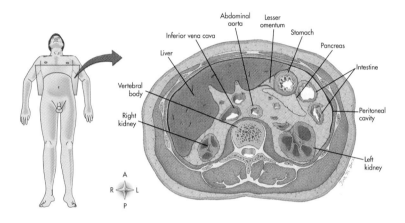

*P*rimary Mechanisms of the Digestive System

Mechanism	Description
Ingestion	Process of taking food into the mouth, starting it on its journey through the digestive tract
Digestion	A group of processes that break complex nutrients into simpler ones, thus facilitating their absorption; *mechanical digestion* physically breaks large chunks into small bits; *chemical digestion* breaks molecules apart
Motility	Movement by the muscular components of the digestive tube, including processes of mechanical digestion; examples include *peristalsis* and *segmentation*
Secretion	Release of digestive juices (containing enzymes, acids, bases, mucus, bile, or other products that facilitate digestion); some digestive organs also secrete endocrine hormones that regulate digestion or metabolism of nutrients
Absorption	Movement of digested nutrients through the GI mucosa and into the internal environment
Elimination	Excretion of the residues of the digestive process (feces) from the rectum, through the anus; defecation

𝒫eristalsis

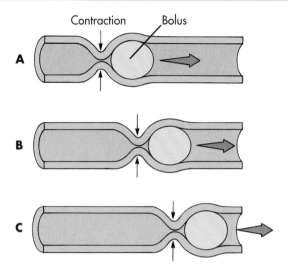

Peristalsis is a progressive type of movement, propelling material from point to point along the GI tract. **A,** A ring of contraction occurs where the GI wall is stretched, pushing the bolus forward. **B,** The moving bolus triggers a ring of contraction in the next region, which pushes the bolus even farther along. **C,** The ring of contraction moves like a wave along the GI tract, pushing the bolus forward.

*S*egmentation

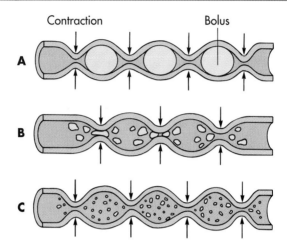

Segmentation is a back-and-forth action that breaks apart chunks of food and mixes in digestive juices. **A,** Ringlike regions of contraction occur at intervals along the GI tract. **B,** Previously contracted regions relax and adjacent regions now contract, effectively "chopping" the contents of each segment into smaller chunks. **C,** Location of the contracted regions continue to alternate back and forth, chopping and mixing the contents of the GI lumen.

Processes of Mechanical Digestion

Organ	Mechanical Process	Nature of Process
Mouth (teeth and tongue)	Mastication	Chewing movements—reduce size of food particles and mix them with saliva
Pharynx	Deglutition	Swallowing—movement of food from mouth to stomach
Esophagus	Deglutition	
	Deglutition	
	Peristalsis	Rippling movements that squeeze food downward in tract; constricted ring forms first in one section, the next, etc., causing waves of contraction to spread along entire canal
Stomach	Churning	Forward and backward movement of gastric contents, mixing food with gastric juices to form chyme
	Peristalsis	Wave starting in body of stomach about three times per minute and sweeping toward closed pyloric sphincter; at intervals, strong peristaltic waves press chyme past sphincter into duodenum
Small intestine	Segmentation (mixing contractions)	Forward and backward movement within segment of intestine; purpose, to mix food and digestive juices thoroughly and to bring all digested food in contact with intestinal mucosa to facilitate absorption; purpose of peristalsis, on the other hand, to propel
	Peristalsis	intestinal contents along digestive tract
Large intestine		
Colon	Segmentation	Churning movements within haustral sacs
	Peristalsis	
Descending colon	Mass peristalsis	Entire contents moved into sigmoid colon and rectum; occurs three or four times a day, usually after a meal
Rectum	Defecation	Emptying of rectum, so-called bowel movement

ℳodel of Digestive Enzyme Action

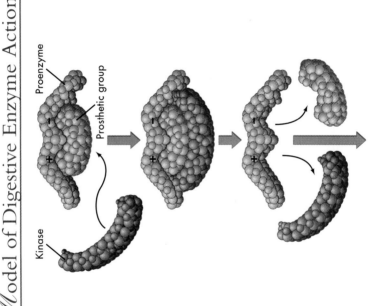

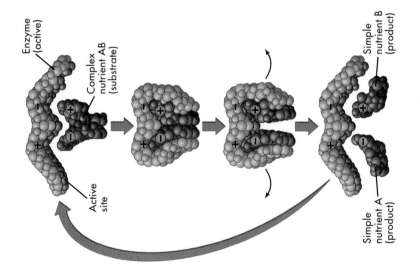

*C*hemical Digestion

Digestive Juices and Enzymes	Substance Digested (or Hydrolyzed)	Resulting Product*
SALIVA		
Amylase	Starch (polysaccharide)	Maltose (a double sugar, or disaccharide)
GASTRIC JUICE		
Protease (pepsin) plus hydrochloric acid	Proteins	Partially digested proteins
PANCREATIC JUICE		
Proteases (e.g., trypsin)†	Proteins (intact or partially digested)	Peptides and amino acids
Lipases	Fats emulsified by bile	Fatty acids, monoglycerides, and glycerol
Amylase	Starch	Maltose
INTESTINAL ENZYMES‡		
Peptidases	Peptides	Amino acids
Sucrase	Sucrose (cane sugar)	Glucose and fructose§ (simple sugars, or monosaccharides)
Lactase	Lactose (milk sugar)	Glucose and galactose (simple sugars)
Maltase	Maltose (malt sugar)	Glucose

*Substances in boldface type are end products of digestion (that is, completely digested nutrients ready for absorption).
†Secreted in inactive form (trypsinogen); activated by enterokinase, an enzyme in the intestinal brush border.
‡Brush-border enzymes.
§Glucose is also called *dextrose*; fructose is also called *levulose*.

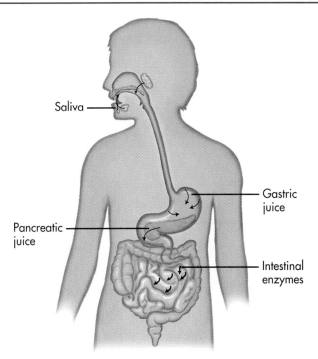

Saliva

Gastric juice

Pancreatic juice

Intestinal enzymes

Acid Secretion by Gastric Parietal Cells

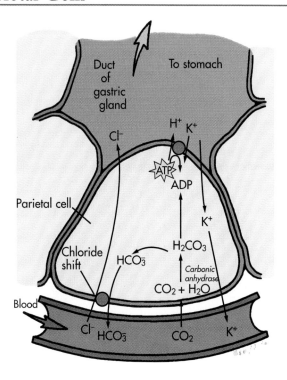

Hydrochloric acid (HCl) secretion by cells of gastric glands uses H^+ produced by the dissociation of carbonic acid (H_2CO_3), which in turn is produced by the reaction of water and carbon dioxide. The chloride (Cl^-) of gastric HCl comes from a chloride shift into the cell in exchange for bicarbonate ions (HCO_3^-) produced by the same dissociation of carbonic acid that yielded the H^+. As Cl^- is shifted into the cell, intracellular Cl^- concentration rises and produces a concentration gradient with the lumen of the gastric gland—forcing Cl^- to diffuse out of the parietal cell. All in all, the net effect is that active pumping of H^+ out of the cell drives the concurrent shift of Cl^- into the cell from the blood and diffusion of Cl^- out of the cell and into the duct of the gastric gland.

Digestive Secretions

Digestive Juice	Source	Substance	Functional Role*
Saliva	Salivary glands	Mucus	*Lubricates bolus of food; facilitates mixing of food*
		Amylase	**Enzyme; begins digestion of starches**
		Sodium bicarbonate	**Increases pH (for optimum amylase function)**
		Water	*Dilutes food and other substances; facilitates mixing*
Gastric juice	Gastric glands	Pepsin	**Enzyme; digests proteins**
		Hydrochloric acid	**Denatures proteins; decreases pH (for optimum pepsin function)**
		Intrinsic factor	**Protects and allows later absorption of vitamin B_{12}**
		Mucus	*Lubricates chyme; protects stomach lining*
		Water	*Dilutes food and other substances; facilitates mixing*
Pancreatic juice	Pancreas (exocrine portion)	Proteases (trypsin, chymo-trypsin, collagenase, elastase, etc.)	**Enzymes; digest proteins and polypeptides**
		Lipases (lipase, phospho-lipase, etc.)	**Enzymes; digest lipids**
		Colipase	**Coenzyme; helps lipase digest fats**
		Nucleases	**Enzymes; digest nucleic acids (RNA and DNA)**
		Amylase	**Enzyme; digests starches**
		Water	*Dilutes food and other substances; facilitates mixing*
		Mucus	*Lubricates*
		Sodium bicarbonate	**Increases pH (for optimum enzyme function)**

Continued

*D*igestive Secretions—cont'd

Digestive Juice	Source	Substance	Functional Role*
Bile	Liver (stored and concentrated in gallbladder)	Lecithin and bile salts	*Emulsify lipids*
		Sodium bicarbonate	**Increases pH (for optimum enzyme function)**
		Cholesterol	Excess cholesterol from body cells, to be excreted with feces
		Products of detoxification	From detoxification of harmful substances by hepatic cells, to be excreted with feces
		Bile pigments (mainly bilirubin)	Products of breakdown of heme groups during hemolysis, to be excreted with feces
		Mucus	Lubrication
		Water	*Dilutes food and other substances; facilitates mixing*
Intestinal juice	Mucosa of small and large intestine	Mucus	Lubrication
		Sodium bicarbonate	**Increases pH (for optimum enzyme function)**
		Water	*Small amount to carry mucus and sodium bicarbonate*

Boldface type indicates a chemical digestive process; *italic type* indicates a mechanical digestive process.

$\mathcal{P}$hases of Gastric Secretion

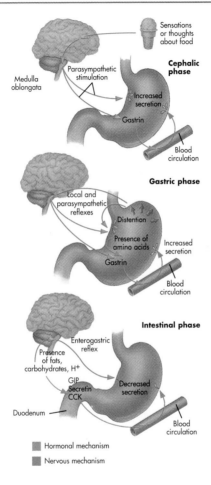

Cephalic phase: Sensations of thoughts about food are relayed to the brainstem, where parasympathetic signals to the gastric mucosa are initiated. This directly stimulates gastric juice secretion and also stimulates the release of gastrin, which prolongs and enhances the effect. *Gastric phase*: The presence of food, specifically the distention it causes, triggers local and parasympathetic nervous reflexes that increase the secretion of gastric juice and gastrin (which further amplifies gastric juice secretion). Products of protein digestion can also trigger the gastrin mechanism. *Intestinal phase*: As food moves into the duodenum, the presence of fats, carbohydrates, and acid stimulates hormonal and nervous reflexes that inhibit stomach activity.

Actions of Some Digestive Hormones Summarized

Hormone	Source	Action
Gastrin	Formed by gastric mucosa in presence of partially digested proteins, when stimulated by the vagus nerve, or when the stomach is stretched	Stimulate secretion of gastric juice rich in pepsin and hydrochloric acid
Gastric inhibitory peptide (GIP)	Formed by intestinal mucosa in presence of fats and perhaps other nutrients	Inhibits gastric secretion and motility
Secretin	Formed by intestinal mucosa in presence of acid, partially digested proteins, and fats	Inhibits gastric secretion; stimulates secretion of pancreatic juice low in enzymes and high in alkalinity (bicarbonate); stimulates ejection of bile by the gallbladder
Cholecystokinin-pancreozymin (CCK)	Formed by intestinal mucosa in presence of fats, partially digested proteins, and acids	Stimulates ejection of bile from gallbladder and secretion of pancreatic juice high in enzymes; opposes the action of gastrin, raising the pH of gastric juice

*I*ntestinal Villus

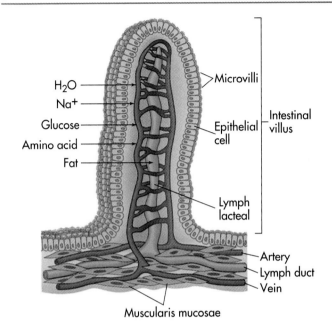

H₂O — Microvilli

Na⁺

Glucose — Epithelial cell

Amino acid

Fat

Intestinal villus

Lymph lacteal

Artery
Lymph duct
Vein

Muscularis mucosae

The presence of intestinal villi and microvilli increases the absorptive surface area of the intestinal mucosa. Most absorbed substances enter the blood in intestinal capillaries, with the exception of fat, which enters lymph by way of the intestinal lacteals.

Absorption of Sodium, Glucose, and Amino Acids

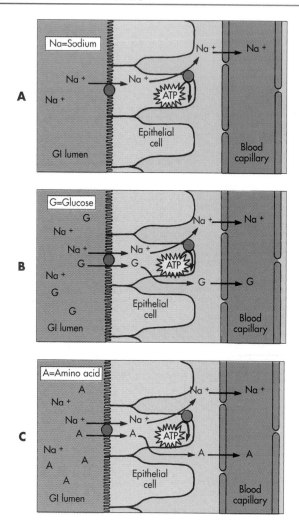

Absorptions of sodium **(A)**, glucose **(B)**, and amino acids **(C)** are all forms of *secondary active transport* because each involves two carriers, one of which is active. The active carrier on the basal side of the epithelial cell maintains a sodium gradient, which facilitates passive transport of sodium, and perhaps another molecule, out of the GI lumen via a passive carrier on the luminal side of the cell.

Absorption of Fats

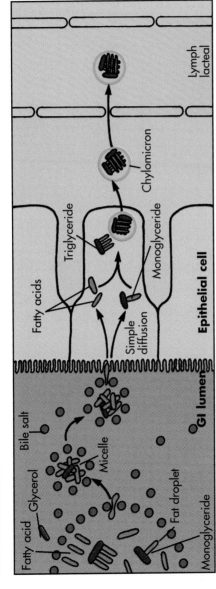

Fats such as triglycerides are chemically digested within emulsified fat droplets, yielding fatty acids, monoglycerides, and glycerol (*left*). Fatty acids and other lipid-soluble compounds (such as cholesterol) leave the fat droplets in small spheres coated with bile salts (micelles). When a micelle reaches the plasma membrane of an absorptive cell, individual fat-soluble molecules diffuse directly into the cytoplasm. The endoplasmic reticulum of the cell resynthesizes fatty acids and monoglycerides into triglycerides. A Golgi body within the cell packages the fats into water-soluble micelles called chylomicrons, which then exit the absorptive cell by exocytosis and enter a lymphatic lacteal.

Summary of Food Absorption Mechanisms

Form Absorbed	Structures into Which Absorbed	Circulation
Protein—as amino acids Perhaps minute quantities of some short-chain polypeptides and whole proteins absorbed, for example, some antibodies	Blood in intestinal capillaries	Portal vein, liver, hepatic vein, inferior vena cava to heart, etc.
Carbohydrates—as simple sugars	Same as amino acids	Same as amino acids
Fats		
Glycerol and monoglycerides	Lymph in intestinal lacteals	During absorption, that is, while in epithelial cells of intestinal mucosa, glycerol and fatty acids recombine to form microscopic packages of fats (chylomicrons); lymphatics carry them by way of thoracic duct to left subclavian vein, superior vena cava, heart, etc.; some fats transported by blood in form of phospholipids or cholesterol esters
Fatty acids combine with bile salts to form water-soluble substance	Lymph in intestinal lacteals	
Some finely emulsified, undigested fats absorbed	Small fraction enters intestinal blood capillaries	

Absorption Sites in the Digestive Tract

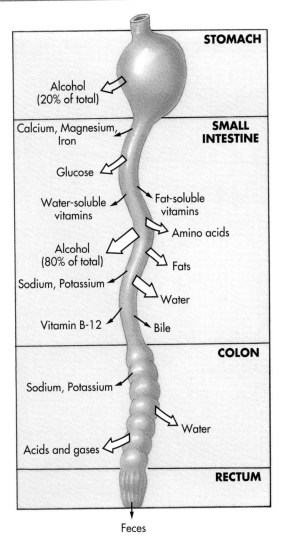

STOMACH

Alcohol
(20% of total)

SMALL INTESTINE

Calcium, Magnesium, Iron

Glucose

Water-soluble vitamins

Fat-soluble vitamins

Amino acids

Alcohol
(80% of total)

Fats

Sodium, Potassium

Water

Vitamin B-12

Bile

COLON

Sodium, Potassium

Water

Acids and gases

RECTUM

Feces

The size of the *arrow* at each site on the illustration above indicates the relative amount of absorption of a particular substance at that site. Notice that most absorption occurs in the intestines, particularly the small intestine.

Summary of Digestive Function

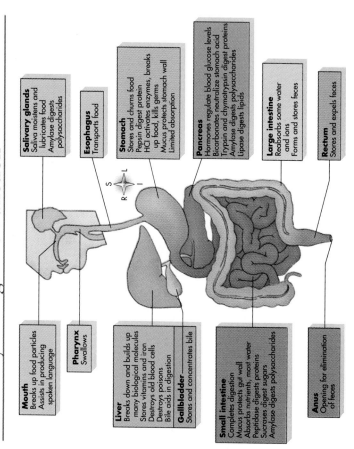

Salivary glands
Saliva moistens and lubricates food
Amylase digests polysaccharides

Esophagus
Transports food

Stomach
Stores and churns food
Pepsin digest protein
HCl activates enzymes, breaks up food, kills germs
Mucus protects stomach wall
Limited absorption

Pancreas
Hormones regulate blood glucose levels
Bicarbonates neutralize stomach acid
Trypsin and chymotrypsin digest proteins
Amylase digests polysaccharides
Lipase digests lipids

Large intestine
Reabsorbs some water and ions
Forms and stores feces

Rectum
Stores and expels feces

Mouth
Breaks up food particles
Assists in producing spoken language

Pharynx
Swallows

Liver
Breaks down and builds up many biological molecules
Stores vitamins and iron
Destroys old blood cells
Destroys poisons
Bile aids in digestion

Gallbladder
Stores and concentrates bile

Small intestine
Completes digestion
Mucus protects gut wall
Absorbs nutrients, most water
Peptidase digests proteins
Sucrases digest sugars
Amylase digests polysaccharides

Anus
Opening for elimination of feces

14

Nutrition and Metabolism

Nutrition refers to the food people eat and the nutrients it contains. Metabolism refers to the complex, interactive set of chemical processes that make life possible. Metabolism is the use the body makes of foods after they have been digested, absorbed, and circulated to the body's cells. The nutrients from food are used by the body as an energy source and as "building blocks" for making complex chemical compounds.

Transferring Chemical Energy

The ability to transfer energy from molecule to molecule is essential to life. The nucleotide adenosine triphosphate (ATP) plays a critical role in transferring energy within living cells. ATP can accept energy from catabolic reactions and transfer that energy to energy-requiring anabolic reactions. Although it is said that ATP is an "energy storage molecule," do not suppose that the energy is stored in the molecule for very long. In fact, an ATP molecule exists for only a brief period before its last phosphate group is broken off and its energy is transferred to another molecule in some metabolic pathway. Long-term storage of energy can be accomplished only by nutrient molecules such as glucose, glycogen, and triglycerides.

In addition to ATP, various other energy-transfer molecules are essential to human life. When atoms in a molecule absorb energy, some of their electrons may move outward to a higher energy level (shell). Electrons often become so energized that they leave the atom completely. As this occurs, pairs of "high-energy" electrons can be picked up and transferred to another molecule by an electron carrier such as flavine adenine dinucleotide (FAD) or nicotinamide adenine dinucleotide (NAD). The illustration below shows how NAD^+ picks up a pair of energized electrons to become NADH. It should be noted here that electrons always travel with a proton (H^+) in metabolic pathways. The electrons do not stay with the electron carrier for long, however. They are immediately transferred to molecules in another metabolic pathway, as the illustration below shows. In the cell, pairs of electrons (and their energy) can thus be transferred from pathway to pathway by NAD and FAD.

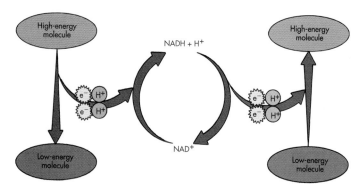

The role of coenzymes in transferring chemical energy.

Glycolysis

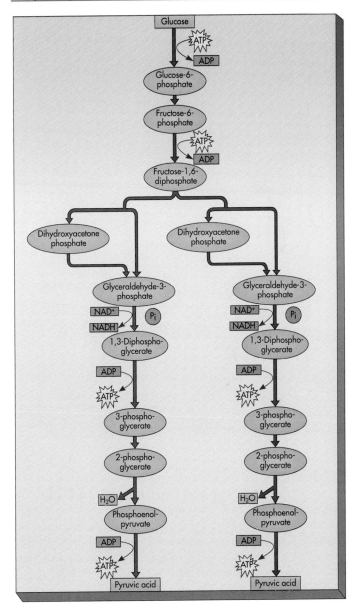

The series of enzyme–catalyzed reactions that make up the portion of the catabolic pathway for carbohydrates called *glycolysis.*

Catabolism of Glucose

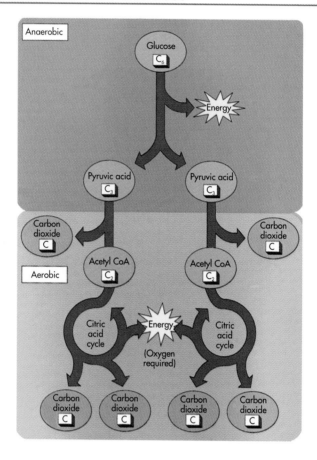

Glycolysis splits one molecule of glucose (six carbon atoms) into two molecules of pyruvic acid (three carbon atoms each). The glycolytic pathway does not require oxygen, so it is termed *anaerobic*. A transition reaction removes a carbon dioxide molecule, converting each pyruvic acid molecule into a two-carbon acetyl group that is escorted by coenzyme A (CoA) into the citric acid cycle. There, two more carbon dioxide molecules (one carbon atom each) are released. The carbon and oxygen atoms in the original glucose molecule are thus released as waste products. However, the real metabolic prize is energy, which is released as the molecule is broken down. Because this part of the pathway requires oxygen, it is termed *aerobic*.

Citric Acid Cycle

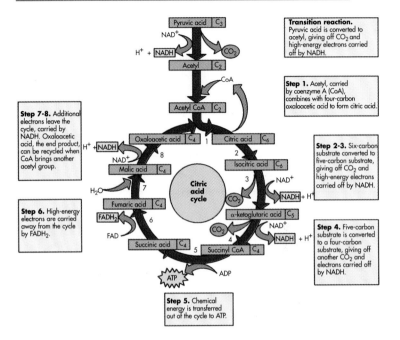

Transition reaction.
Pyruvic acid is converted to acetyl, giving off CO_2 and high-energy electrons carried off by NADH.

Step 1. Acetyl, carried by coenzyme A (CoA), combines with four-carbon oxaloacetic acid to form citric acid.

Step 2-3. Six-carbon substrate converted to five-carbon substrate, giving off CO_2 and high-energy electrons carried off by NADH.

Step 4. Five-carbon substrate is converted to a four-carbon substrate, giving off another CO_2 and electrons carried off by NADH.

Step 5. Chemical energy is transferred out of the cycle to ATP.

Step 6. High-energy electrons are carried away from the cycle by $FADH_2$.

Step 7-8. Additional electrons leave the cycle, carried by NADH. Oxaloacetic acid, the end product, can be recycled when CoA brings another acetyl group.

Each pyruvic acid molecule is prepared to enter the citric acid cycle by the transition reaction, which yields a pair of high-energy electrons and a CO_2 molecule. The acetyl group that is thus formed is picked up by coenzyme A (*CoA*) and led into the citric acid cycle proper, which is described here as a recurring series of eight steps.

*E*lectron Transport System

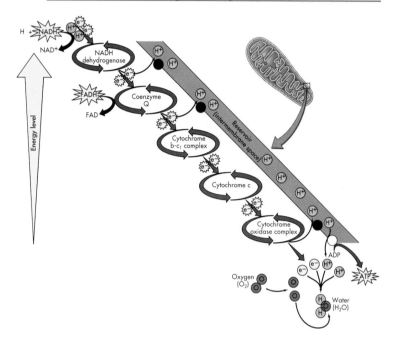

Pairs of high-energy electrons and their accompanying protons (H$^+$) are transferred to the components (cytochromes) of the electron transport system by NAD and FAD. They then jump from cytochrome to cytochrome, losing energy along the way. The energy is used to pump protons (H^+) into the compartment between the inner and outer mitochondrial membranes. The diffusion of protons back into the inner compartment drives the phosphorylation of adenosine diphosphate (ADP) to form ATP. The protons are joined with oxygen and low-energy electrons at the end of the cytochrome chain to form water molecules. This all takes place within each mitochondrion.

$\mathscr{E}$nergy Extracted From Glucose

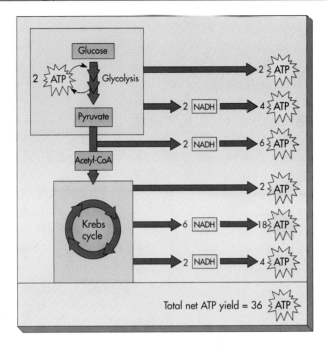

Energy freed in the breakdown of glucose is released mostly as heat, but some of it is transferred to a usable form—the high-energy bonds of ATP. In most human cells, one glucose molecule produces enough usable chemical energy to synthesize or "charge up" 36 ATP molecules. Some cells, such as heart and liver cells, shuttle electrons more efficiently and may be able to synthesize up to 38 ATP molecules. This represents an energy conversion efficiency of 38% to 44%, much better than the 20% to 25% typical of most machines.

*S*ummary of Glucose Metabolism

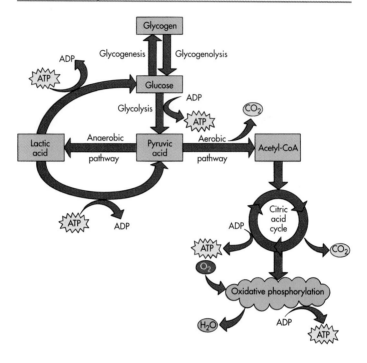

Glucose is catabolized to pyruvic acid in the process of glycolysis. If oxygen is available, pyruvic acid is converted to acetyl-CoA and then enters the citric acid cycle and transfers energy to the maximum number of ATP molecules via oxidative phosphorylation. If oxygen is not available, pyruvic acid is converted to lactic acid, incurring an oxygen debt. The oxygen debt is later repaid when ATP produced via oxidative phosphorylation is used to convert lactic acid back into pyruvic acid or all the way back to glucose. If there is an excess of glucose, the cell may convert it to glycogen (glycogenesis). Later, individual glucose molecules can be removed from the glycogen chain by the process of glycogenolysis. Although NAD and FAD play important roles in these pathways, they have been left out of this diagram for the sake of simplicity.

Hormonal Control of Blood Glucose Level

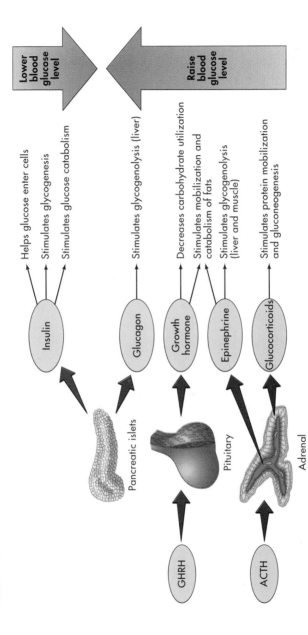

Insulin lowers blood glucose level and is therefore hypoglycemic. Most hormones raise blood glucose level and are called hyperglycemic, or anti-insulin, hormones.

Amino Acids

Essential (Indispensible)	Nonessential (Dispensable)
Histidine*	Alanine
Isoleucine	Arginine
Leucine	Asparagine
Lysine	Aspartic acid
Methionine	Cysteine
Phenylalanine	Glutamic acid
Threonine	Glutamine
Tryptophan	Glycine
Valine	Proline
	Serine
	Tyrosine†

*Essential in infants and, perhaps, adult males.
†Can be synthesized from phenylalanine; therefore is nonessential as long as phenylalanine is in the diet.

*S*ummary of Metabolism

Nutrient	Anabolism	Catabolism
Carbohydrates	Temporary excess changed into glycogen by liver cells in presence of insulin; stored in liver and skeletal muscles until needed and then changed back to glucose	Oxidized, in presence of insulin, to yield energy (4.1 kcal per g) and wastes (carbon dioxide and water)
	True excess beyond body's energy requirements converted into adipose tissue; stored in various fat depots of body	$C_6H_{12}O6 + 6\ O_2 \rightarrow$ Energy $+ 6\ CO_2 + 6\ H_2O$
Fats	Built into adipose tissue; stored in fat depots of body	Fatty acids $\rightarrow$ Glycerol $\rightarrow$ (glycolysis) (beta–oxidation) Acetyl–CoA
		Acetyl–CoA $\leftrightarrows$ Ketones (tissues; citric acid cycle) $\rightarrow$ Energy (9.3 kcal per g) $+ CO_2 + H_2O$
Proteins	Synthesized into tissue proteins, blood proteins, enzymes, hormones, etc.	Deaminated by liver, forming ammonia (which is converted to urea) and keto acids (which are either oxidized or changed to glucose or fat)

*S*ummary of Metabolism—cont'd

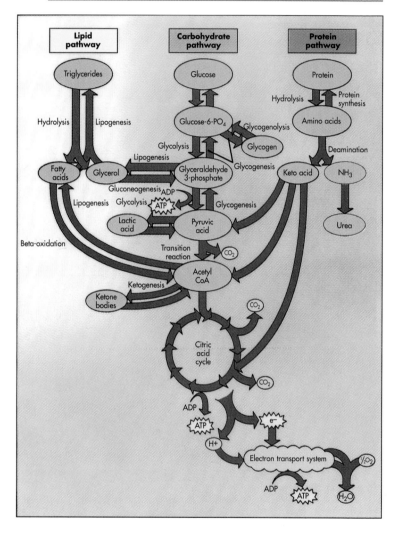

Notice the central role played by the citric acid cycle and electron transport system. Notice also how different molecules can be converted to forms that may enter other pathways.

Major Vitamins

Vitamin	Dietary Source	Functions	Symptoms of Deficiency
Vitamin A	Green and yellow vegetables, dairy products, and liver	Maintains epithelial tissue and produces visual pigments	Night blindness and flaking skin
B-complex vitamins			
B₁ (thiamine)	Grains, meat, and legumes	Helps enzymes in the citric acid cycle	Nerve problems (beriberi), heart muscle weakness, and edema
B₂ (riboflavin)	Green vegetables, organ meats, eggs, and dairy products	Aids enzymes in the citric acid cycle	Inflammation of skin and eyes
B₃ (niacin)	Meat and grains	Helps enzymes in the citric acid cycle	Pellagra (scaly dermatitis and mental disturbances) and nervous disorders
B₅ (pantothenic acid)	Organ meat, eggs, and liver	Aids enzymes that connect fat and carbohydrate metabolism	Loss of coordination (rare)
B₆ (pyridoxine)	Vegetables, meats, and grains	Helps enzymes that catabolize amino acids	Convulsions, irritability, and anemia

Continued

*M*ajor Vitamins—cont'd

Vitamin	Dietary Source	Functions	Symptoms of Deficiency
B$_9$ (folic acid)	Vegetables	Aids enzymes in amino acid catabolism and blood production	Digestive disorders and anemia
B$_{12}$ (cyanocobalamin)	Meat and dairy products	Involved in blood production and other processes	Pernicious anemia
Biotin (vitamin H)	Vegetables, meat, and eggs	Helps enzymes in amino acid catabolism and fat and glycogen synthesis	Mental and muscle problems (rare)
Vitamin C (ascorbic acid)	Fruits and green vegetables	Helps in manufacture of collagen fibers; antioxidant	Scurvy and degeneration of skin, bone, and blood vessels
Vitamin D (calciferol)	Dairy products and fish liver oil	Aids in calcium absorption	Rickets and skeletal deformity
Vitamin E (tocopherol)	Green vegetables and seeds	Protects cell membranes from being destroyed	Muscle and reproductive disorders (rare)

*M*ajor Minerals

Mineral	Dietary Source	Functions	Symptoms of Deficiency
Calcium (Ca)	Dairy products, legumes, and vegetables	Helps blood clotting, bone formation, and nerve and muscle function	Bone degeneration and nerve and muscle malfunction
Chlorine (Cl)	Salty foods	Aids in stomach acid production and acid-base balance	Acid-base imbalance
Cobalt (Co)	Meat	Helps vitamin B_{12} in blood cell production	Pernicious anemia
Copper (Cu)	Seafood, organ meats, and legumes	Involved in extracting energy from the citric acid cycle and in blood production	Fatigue and anemia
Iodine (I)	Seafood and iodized salt	Required for thyroid hormone synthesis	Goiter (thyroid enlargement) and decrease of metabolic rate
Iron (Fe)	Meat, eggs, vegetables, and legumes	Involved in extracting energy from the citric acid cycle and in blood production	Fatigue and anemia
Magnesium (Mg)	Vegetables and grains	Helps many enzymes	Nerve disorders, blood vessel dilation, and heart rhythm problems
Manganese (Mn)	Vegetables, legumes, and grains	Helps many enzymes	Muscle and nerve disorders
Phosphorus (P)	Dairy products and meat	Aids in bone formation and is used to make ATP, DNA, RNA, and phospholipids	Bone degeneration and metabolic problems
Potassium (K)	Seafood, milk, fruit, and meats	Helps muscle and nerve function	Muscle weakness, heart problems, and nerve problems
Sodium (Na)	Salty foods	Aids in muscle and nerve function and fluid balance	Weakness and digestive upset
Zinc (Zn)	Many foods	Helps many enzymes	Inadequate growth

45

Urinary System

The principal organs of the urinary system are the kidneys, which process blood and form urine as a waste to be excreted (removed from the body). The excreted urine travels from the kidney to the outside of the body via accessory organs: ureters, urinary bladder, and urethra.

Location of the Urinary System Organs

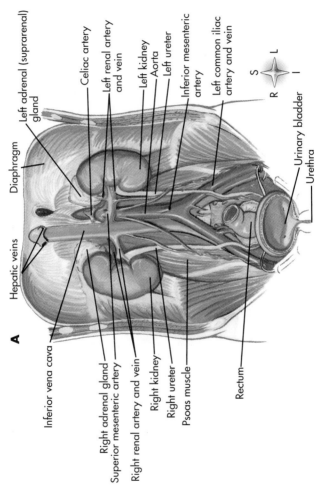

A, Anterior view of urinary organs with the peritoneum and visceral organs removed. *Continued*

*L*ocation of the Urinary System Organs—cont'd

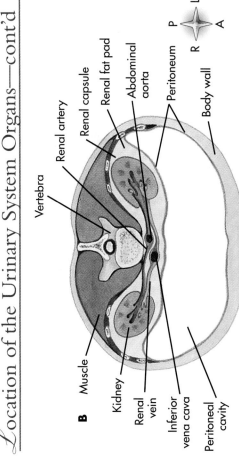

B

Vertebra

Renal artery

Renal capsule

Renal fat pad

Abdominal aorta

Peritoneum

Body wall

Muscle

Kidney

Renal vein

Inferior vena cava

Peritoneal cavity

P

R — L

A

B, Horizontal (transverse) section of the abdomen showing the retroperitoneal position of the kidneys.

Internal Structure of the Kidney

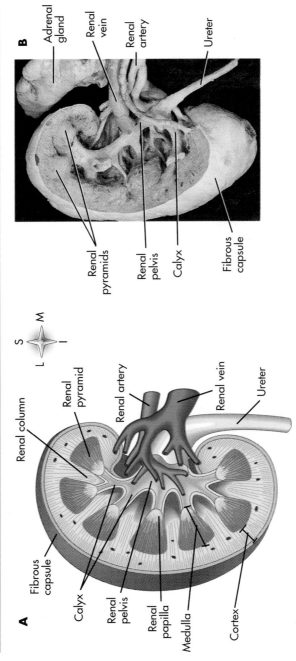

Coronal section of the right kidney in an artist's rendering, **A**, and in a photograph of a preserved human kidney, **B**.

Circulation of Blood Through the Kidney

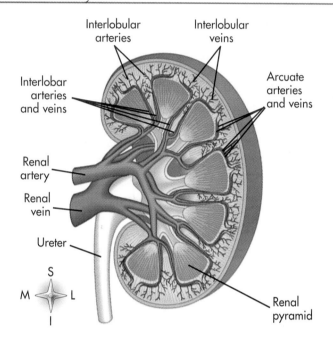

This illustration shows the major arteries and veins of the renal circulation.

$\mathcal{N}$ephron

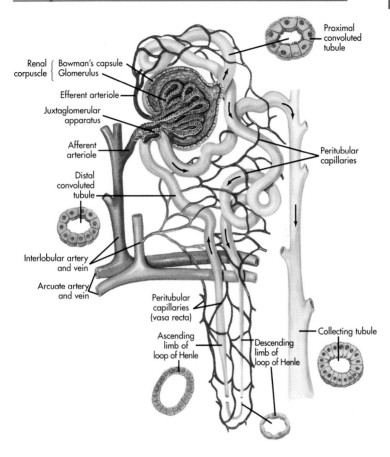

Proximal convoluted tubule

Renal corpuscle { Bowman's capsule
Glomerulus

Efferent arteriole

Juxtaglomerular apparatus

Afferent arteriole

Peritubular capillaries

Distal convoluted tubule

Interlobular artery and vein

Arcuate artery and vein

Peritubular capillaries (vasa recta)

Ascending limb of loop of Henle

Descending limb of loop of Henle

Collecting tubule

The nephron is the base functional unit of the kidney. This illustration of a single nephron unit also shows the surrounding peritubular blood vessels.

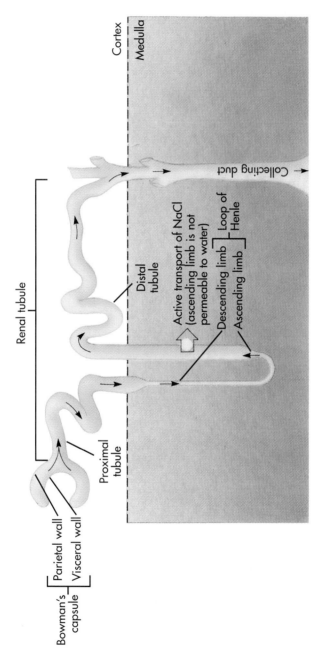

Schematic diagram showing the essential components of a nephron. *Arrows* indicate direction of flow of fluid within the tubule.

Structure of the Urinary Bladder

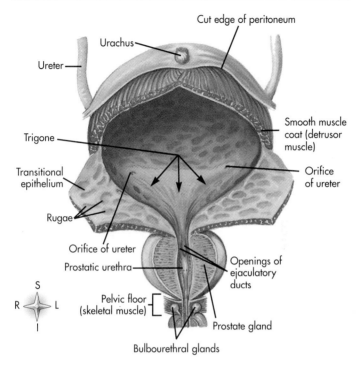

Frontal view of a dissected urinary bladder (male) in a fully distended position.

*L*ocation of the Urinary Bladder

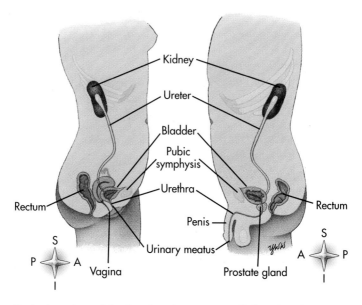

Kidney
Ureter
Bladder
Pubic symphysis
Urethra
Penis
Rectum
Rectum
S
S
P
A
A
P
I
I
Urinary meatus
Vagina
Prostate gland

Sagittal section of the female urinary system (*left*) and male urinary system (*right*), each showing a partially distended bladder.

ℒocation of the Nephron

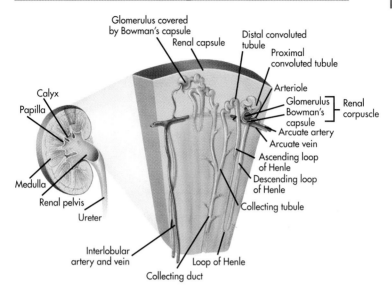

Magnified wedge shows that renal corpuscles (Bowman's capsules with invaginated glomeruli) and both proximal and distal convoluted tubules are located in the cortex of the kidney. The medulla contains loops of Henle and collecting tubules. The blood vessel that brings blood to the glomerulus (afferent arteriole) has a larger diameter than the blood vessel that drains blood from it (efferent arteriole).

*M*echanism of Urine Formation

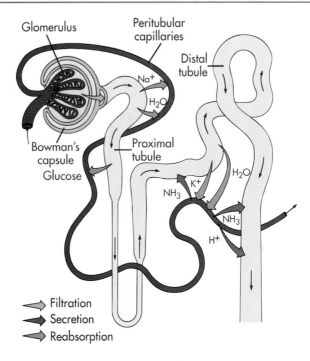

Diagram shows the mechanisms of urine formation and where they occur in the nephron:

1. *Filtration,* or the movement of water and solutes from the plasma in the glomerulus, across the glomerular-capsular membrane, and into the capsular space of the Bowman's capsule.
2. *Reabsorption,* or the movement of molecules out of the tubule and into the peritubular blood.
3. *Secretion,* or the movement of molecules out of the peritubular blood and into the tubule for excretion.

Forces Affecting Glomerular Filtration

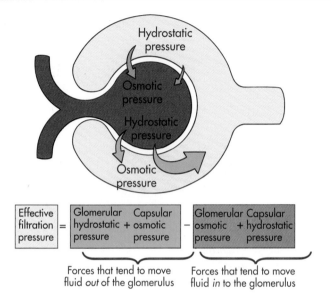

Effective filtration pressure	=	Glomerular hydrostatic pressure + Capsular osmotic pressure	−	Glomerular osmotic pressure + Capsular hydrostatic pressure

Forces that tend to move fluid *out* of the glomerulus

Forces that tend to move fluid *in* to the glomerulus

Effective filtration pressure (EFP) is determined by comparing the forces that push fluid into the capillary with those that push it out of the capillary.

*M*echanisms of Tubular Reabsorption

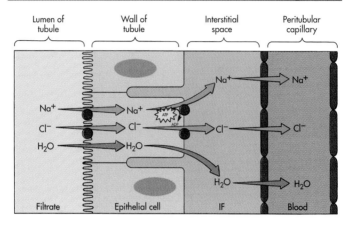

Sodium ions (Na^+) are pumped from tubule cell to interstitial fluid (*IF*), increasing interstitial Na^+ concentration to a level that drives the diffusion of Na^+ into blood. As Na^+ is pumped out of the cell, more Na^+ passively diffuses in from filtrate to maintain an equilibrium of concentration. Enough Na^+ moves out of the tubule and into blood that an electrical gradient is established (blood is positive relative to filtrate). Electrical attraction between oppositely charged particles drives the diffusion of negative ions in filtrate, such as chloride (Cl^-), into blood. As the ion concentration in blood increases, osmosis of water from the tubule occurs. Thus active transport of sodium creates a situation that promotes passive transport of negative ions and water.

$\mathcal{T}$he Countercurrent Multiplier System in the Loop of Henle

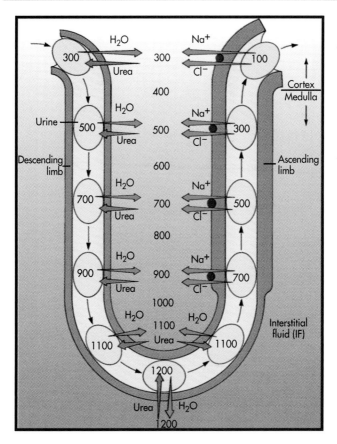

Na^+ and Cl^- are pumped from the ascending limb and moved into interstitial fluid (*IF*) to maintain a high osmolality there. Because salt content of the medullary IF increases, this is called a "multiplier" mechanism. Because ion pumping also lowers the tubule fluid's osmolality by 200 mOsm, fluid leaving the loop of Henle is only 100 mOsm (hypotonic), compared to 300 mOsm (isotonic) when it entered the loop. Numbers in the diagram are expressed in milliosmoles.

The Countercurrent Exchange Mechanism in the Vasa Recta

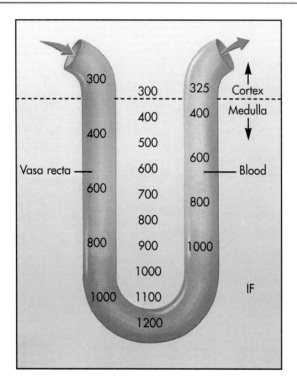

Because the vasa recta forms a countercurrent loop, blood leaving the capillary bed has only a slightly higher solute content than when it entered. Thus high osmolality of medullary tissue fluid is maintained. If peritubular blood instead traveled straight through the tissue, all excess solute in the medulla would be removed, and the osmolality of medullary interstitial fluid would be equivalent to that of the cortex. Numbers in the diagram are expressed in milliosmoles.

Production of Hypotonic Urine

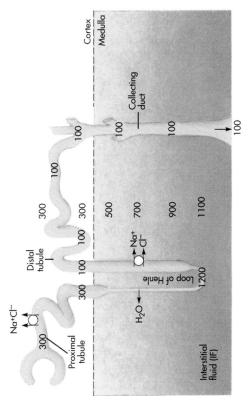

Hypotonic urine is produced by the nephron through the mechanism shown here. Isotonic (300 mOsm) tubule fluid that enters the loop of Henle becomes hypotonic (100 mOsm) by the time it enters the distal tubule. The tubule fluid remains hypotonic as it is conducted out of the kidney because the walls of the distal tubule and collecting duct are impermeable to H_2O, Na^+, and Cl^-. Values are expressed in milliosmoles.

*P*roduction of Hypertonic Urine

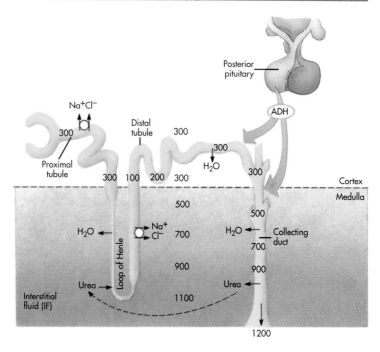

Hypertonic urine can be formed when ADH is present. ADH, a posterior pituitary hormone, increases the water permeability of the distal tubule and collecting duct. Thus hypotonic (100 mOsm) tubule fluid leaving the loop of Henle can equilibrate first with the isotonic (300 mOsm) interstitial fluid (*IF*) of the cortex, then with the increasingly hypertonic (400 to 1,200 mOsm) IF of the medulla. As H_2O leaves the collecting duct by osmosis, the filtrate becomes more concentrated with solutes left behind. The concentration gradient causes urea to diffuse into the IF, where some of it is eventually picked up by tubule fluid in the descending limb of the loop of Henle (*dashed line*). This countercurrent movement of urea helps maintain high solute concentration in the medulla. Values are expressed in milliosmoles.

Summary of Nephron Function

Part of Nephron	Function	Substance Moved
Renal corpuscle	Filtration (passive)	Water
		Smaller solute particles (ions, glucose, etc.)
Proximal tubule	Reabsorption (active)	Active transport: Na^+
		Cotransport: glucose and amino acids
	Reabsorption (passive)	Diffusion: Cl^-, $PO_4^=$, urea, other solutes
		Osmosis: water
Loop of Henle		
Descending limb	Reabsorption (passive)	Osmosis: water
	Secretion (passive)	Diffusion: urea
Ascending limb	Reabsorption (active)	Active transport: Na^+
	Reabsorption (passive)	Diffusion: Cl^-
Distal tubule	Reabsorption (active)	Active transport: Na^+
	Reabsorption (passive)	Diffusion: Cl^-, other anions
		Osmosis: water (only in presence of ADH)
	Secretion (passive)	Diffusion: ammonia
	Secretion (active)	Active transport: K^+, H^+, some drugs
Collecting duct	Reabsorption (active)	Active transport: Na^+
	Reabsorption (passive)	Diffusion: urea
		Osmosis: water (only in presence of ADH)
	Secretion (passive)	Diffusion: ammonia
	Secretion (active)	Active transport: K^+, H^+, some drugs

Characteristics of Urine

Normal Characteristics	Abnormal Characteristics
COLOR	
Transparent yellow, amber, or straw color	Abnormal colors or cloudiness, which may indicate presence of blood, bile, bacteria, drugs, food pigments, or high-solute concentration
COMPOUNDS	
Mineral ions (for example, Na^+, Cl^-, K^+)	Acetone
Nitrogenous wastes: ammonia, creatinine, urea, uric acid	Albumin Bile
Suspended solids (sediment)*: bacteria, blood cells, casts (solid matter)	Glucose
Urine pigments	
ODOR	
Slight odor	Acetone odor, which is common in diabetes mellitus
pH	
4.6–8.0 (freshly voided urine is generally acidic)	High in alkalosis; low in acidosis
SPECIFIC GRAVITY	
1.001–1.035	High specific gravity can cause precipitation of solutes and formation of kidney stones

*Occasional trace amounts.

$\mathscr{U}$rine Components

Test	Normal Values*	Significance of a Change
ROUTINE URINALYSIS		
Acetone and acetoacetate	0	↑ during fasting ↑ in diabetic acidosis
Albumin	0–trace	↑ in hypertension ↑ in kidney disease ↑ after strenuous exercise (temporary)
Ammonia	20–70 mEq/L	↑ in liver disease ↑ in diabetes mellitus
Bile and bilirubin	—	↑ during obstruction of the bile ducts
Calcium	<150 mg/day	↑ in hyperparathyroidism ↓ in hypoparathyroidism
Color	Transparent yellow, straw-colored, or amber	Abnormal color or cloudiness may indicate blood in urine, bile, bacteria, drugs, food pigments, or high solute concentration
Odor	Characteristic slight odor	Acetone odor in diabetes mellitus (diabetic ketosis)
Osmolality	500–800 mOsm/L	↑ in dehydration ↑ in heart failure ↓ in diabetes insipidus ↓ in aldosteronism

Continued

*U*rine Components—cont'd

Test	Normal Values*	Significance of a Change
ROUTINE URINALYSIS—cont'd		
pH	4.6–8.0	↑ in alkalosis ↑ during urinary infections → in acidosis → in dehydration → in emphysema
Potassium	25–100 mEq/L	↑ in dehydration ↑ in chronic kidney failure → in diarrhea or vomiting → in adrenal insufficiency
Sodium	75–200 mg/day	↑ in starvation ↑ in dehydration → in acute kidney failure → in Cushing's syndrome
Creatinine clearance	100–140 ml/min	↑ in kidney disease
Creatine	1–2 g/day	↑ in infections → in some kidney diseases → in anemia (some forms)
Glucose	0	↑ in diabetes mellitus ↑ in hyperthyroidism ↑ in hypersecretion of adrenal cortex
Urea clearance	>40 ml blood cleared per min	↑ in some kidney diseases

Urea	25–35 g/day	↑ in some liver diseases
		↑ in hemolytic anemia
		↓ during obstruction of bile ducts
		↓ in severe diarrhea
Uric acid	0.6–1.0 g/day	↑ in gout
		↓ in some kidney diseases
MICROSCOPIC EXAMINATION		
Bacteria	<10,000/ml	↑ during urinary infections
Blood cells (RBC)	0–trace	↑ in pyelonephritis
		↑ from damage by calculi
		↑ in infection
		↑ in cancer
Blood cells (WBC)	0–trace	↑ in infections
Blood cell casts (RBC)	0–trace	↑ in pyelonephritis
Blood cell casts (WBC)	0–trace	↑ in infection
Crystals	0–trace	↑ in urinary retention
		Very large crystaline masses are calculi.
Epithelial casts	0–trace	↑ in some kidney disorders
		↑ in heavy metal toxicity
Granular casts	0–trace	↑ in some kidney disorders
Hyaline casts	0–trace	↑ in some kidney disorders
		↑ in fever

*Values vary with the analysis method used.

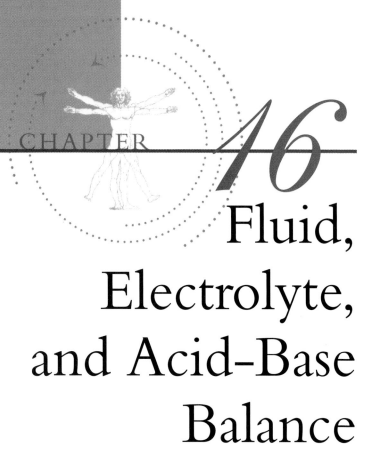

CHAPTER 16

Fluid, Electrolyte, and Acid–Base Balance

The volume of fluid and the electrolyte levels inside the cells, in the interstitial spaces, and in the blood vessels all remain relatively constant when a condition of homeostasis exists. Fluid and electrolyte imbalance, then, means that both the total volume of water or level of electrolytes in the body or the amounts in one or more of its fluid compartments have increased or decreased beyond normal limits.

Acid–base balance refers to regulation of hydrogen ion concentration (pH) in the body fluids. Precise regulation of pH at the cellular level is necessary for survival. Even slight deviations from normal pH will result in pronounced, potentially fatal changes in metabolic activity.

Distribution of Total Body Water

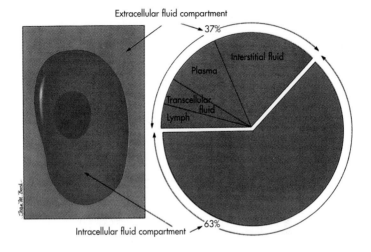

Functionally, the total body water can be subdivided into two major fluid compartments called the *extracellular* and the *intracellular* fluid compartments. Extracellular fluid (ECF) consists mainly of the plasma found in the blood vessels and the interstitial fluid that surrounds the cells. In addition, the lymph and so-called *transcellular fluid*—such as cerebrospinal fluid and the specialized joint fluids—are also considered as ECF. Intracellular fluid (ICF) refers to the water inside the cells.

ECF constitutes the internal environment of the body. It therefore serves the dual vital functions of providing a relatively constant environment for cells and of transporting substances to and from them. ICF, on the other hand, because it is a solvent, functions to facilitate intracellular chemical reactions that maintain life.

$\mathscr{R}$elative Volumes of Three Body Fluids

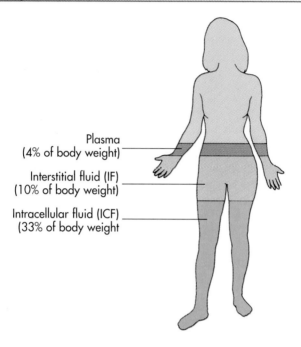

Plasma
(4% of body weight)

Interstitial fluid (IF)
(10% of body weight)

Intracellular fluid (ICF)
(33% of body weight

Values shown here represent the typical normal fluid distribution in a young adult.

$\mathscr{V}$olumes of Body Fluid Compartments*

Body Fluid	Infant	Adult Male	Adult Female
EXTRACELLULAR FLUID			
Plasma	4	4	4
Interstitial fluid	26	15	10
INTRACELLULAR FLUID	45	38	33
TOTAL	75	57	47

*Percentage of body weight.

Chief Chemical Constituents
of Three Fluid Compartments

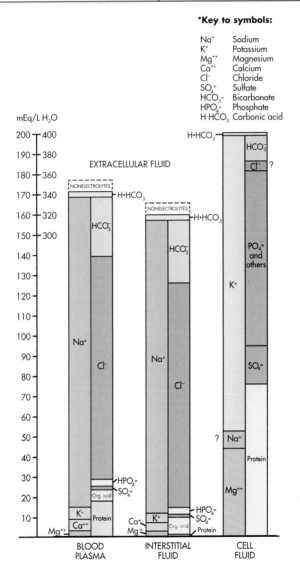

*Key to symbols:

Na^+	Sodium
K^+	Potassium
Mg^{++}	Magnesium
Ca^{++}	Calcium
Cl^-	Chloride
$SO_4^=$	Sulfate
HCO_3^-	Bicarbonate
$HPO_4^=$	Phosphate
$H\cdot HCO_3$	Carbonic acid

The column of figures at the *left* (200, 190, 180, etc.) indicates amounts of cation or of anion, whereas the figures on the *right* (400, 380, 360, etc.) indicate the sum of the cations and anions.

$\mathcal{T}$ypical Normal Values for Each Portal of Water Entry and Exit (With Wide Variations)

Intake		Output	
Water in foods	700 ml	Lungs (water in expired air)	350 ml
Ingested liquids	1,500 ml	Skin	
Water formed by catabolism	200 ml	By diffusion	350 ml
		By sweat	100 ml
		Kidneys (urine)	1,400 ml
		Intestines (in feces)	200 ml
TOTALS	2,400 ml		2,400 ml

$\mathcal{M}$echanisms of Fluid and Electrolyte Regulation

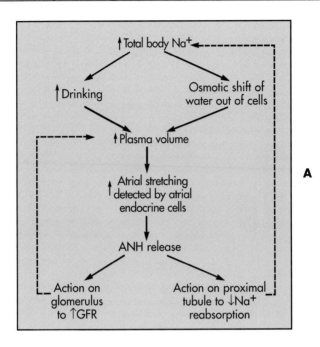

A

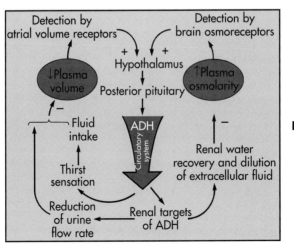

B

A, The atrial natriuretic hormone (ANH) system. **B,** The antidiuretic hormone (ADH) system. *Continued*

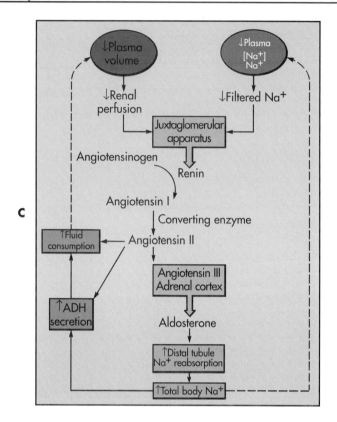

C, The aldosterone system.

The Effects of Dehydration

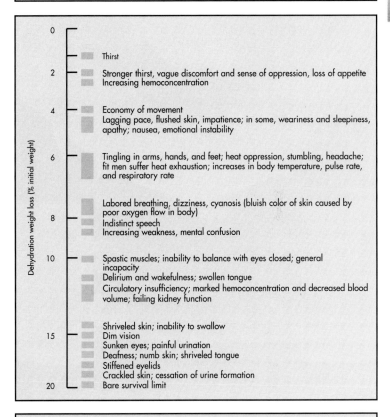

NORMAL WEIGHT

Dehydration weight loss (% initial weight)

- 0
- Thirst
- 2 — Stronger thirst, vague discomfort and sense of oppression, loss of appetite
  Increasing hemoconcentration
- 4 — Economy of movement
  Lagging pace, flushed skin, impatience; in some, weariness and sleepiness,
  apathy; nausea, emotional instability
- 6 — Tingling in arms, hands, and feet; heat oppression, stumbling, headache;
  fit men suffer heat exhaustion; increases in body temperature, pulse rate,
  and respiratory rate

  Labored breathing, dizziness, cyanosis (bluish color of skin caused by
  poor oxygen flow in body)
- 8 — Indistinct speech
  Increasing weakness, mental confusion
- 10 — Spastic muscles; inability to balance with eyes closed; general
  incapacity
  Delirium and wakefulness; swollen tongue
  Circulatory insufficiency; marked hemoconcentration and decreased blood
  volume; failing kidney function

  Shriveled skin; inability to swallow
- 15 — Dim vision
  Sunken eyes; painful urination
  Deafness; numb skin; shriveled tongue
  Stiffened eyelids
  Crackled skin; cessation of urine formation
- 20 — Bare survival limit

DEATH

Donnan Equilibrium

According to the Donnan equilibrium principle, when nondiffusible anions (negative ions) are present on one side of a membrane, there are on that side of the membrane fewer diffusible anions and more diffusible cations (positive ions) than on the other side. Applying this principle to the blood and interstitial fluid, it is reasoned that because blood contains nondiffusible protein anions, it contains fewer chloride ions (diffusible anions) and more sodium ions (diffusible cations) than does interstitial fluid.

*M*ovement of Fluids and Electrolytes

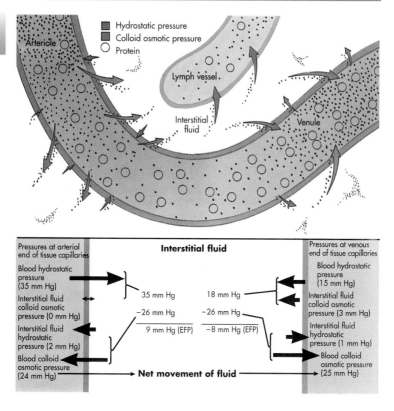

The illustration above shows the movement of fluids and electrolytes between plasma and interstitial fluid caused by hydrostatic and colloid and osmotic pressure.

*M*echanisms of Edema Formation in Some Common Conditions

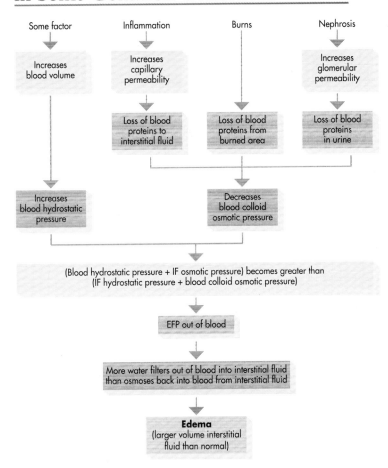

IF, Interstitial fluid; *EFP*, effective or net filtration pressure.

ℋow Electrolyte Imbalance Leads to Fluid Imbalances

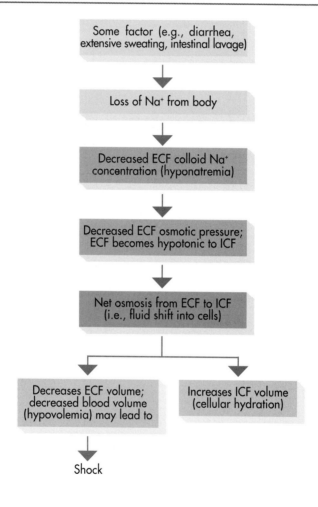

The schematic above uses the example of sodium deficit (hyponatremia) and resulting hypovolemia (cellular hydration). *ECF,* Extracellular fluid; *ICF,* intracellular fluid.

Antidiuretic Hormone (ADH) Mechanism for ECF Homeostasis

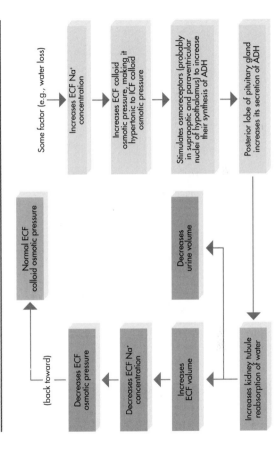

Some factor (e.g., water loss)

Increases ECF Na$^+$ concentration

Increases ECF colloid osmotic pressure, making it hypertonic to ICF colloid osmotic pressure

Stimulates osmoreceptors (probably in supraoptic and paraventricular nuclei of hypothalamus) to increase their synthesis of ADH

Posterior lobe of pituitary gland increases its secretion of ADH

Increases kidney tubule reabsorption of water

Decreases urine volume

Increases ECF volume

Decreases ECF Na$^+$ concentration

Decreases ECF osmotic pressure

(back toward)

Normal ECF colloid osmotic pressure

The ADH mechanism helps maintain homeostasis of ECF colloid osmotic pressure by regulating its volume and thereby its electrolyte concentration, that is, mainly ECF Na$^+$ concentration.

The pH Range

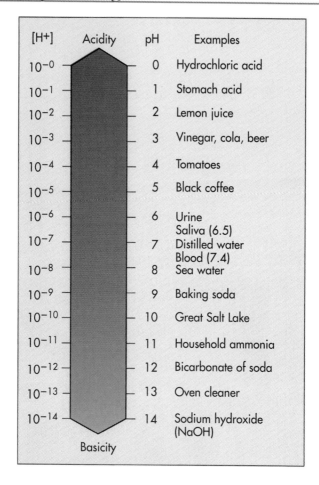

The pH value is shown on the right side of the scale and the corresponding logarithmic value is on the left.

*p*H Control Systems

Type	Response Time	Example
Chemical buffer systems	Rapid	Bicarbonate buffer system Phosphate buffer system Protein buffer system
Physiological buffer systems	Delayed	Respiratory response system Renal response system

*I*ntegration of pH Control Mechanisms

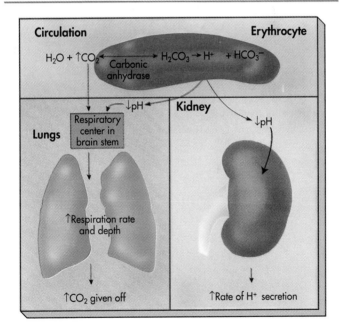

Elevated CO_2 levels result in increased formation of carbonic acid in red blood cells (RBCs). The resulting increase in hydrogen ions, coupled with elevated CO_2 levels, results in an increase in respiratory rate and secretion of hydrogen ions by the kidneys, thus helping to regulate the pH of body fluids.

$\mathscr{B}$uffering Action of Sodium Bicarbonate

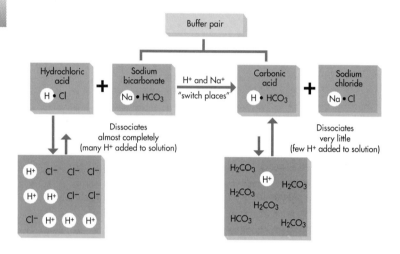

Buffering of acid HCl by NaHCO$_3$. As a result of the buffer action, the strong acid (HCl) is replaced by a weaker acid (H · HCO$_3$). Note that HCl, as a strong acid, "dissociates" almost completely and releases more H$^+$ than H$_2$CO$_3$. Buffering decreases the number of H$^+$ ions in the system.

$\mathscr{B}$uffering Action of Carbonic Acid

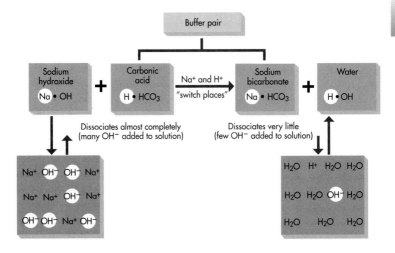

Buffering of base NaOH by H_2CO_3. As a result of buffer action, the strong base (NaOH) is replaced by H_2CO_3 and H_2O. As a strong base, NaOH "dissociates" almost completely and releases large quantities of OH^-. Dissociation of H_2O is minimal. Buffering decreases the number of OH^- in the system.

Chloride Shift

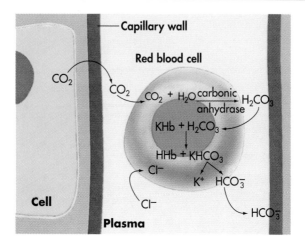

Concentration of chloride ions (Cl^-) in RBCs increases as bicarbonate ions (HCO_3^-) diffuse out of the cell. Bicarbonate ions form as a result of the buffering of carbonic acid by the potassium salt of hemoglobin.

Mechanisms That Control Urine pH

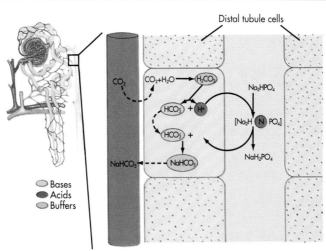

Acidification of urine and conservation of base by distal renal tubule excretion of H^+. A decrease in blood pH accelerates the renal tubule ion-exchange mechanisms that acidify urine and conserve blood's base, thereby tending to increase blood pH back to normal. Distal and collecting tubules secrete hydrogen ions into the urine in exchange for basic ions, which they reabsorb. Note in the figure that carbon dioxide diffuses from tubule capillaries into distal tubule cells, where the enzyme carbonic anhydrase accelerates the combining of carbon dioxide with water to form carbonic acid. The carbonic acid dissociates into hydrogen ions and bicarbonate ions. The hydrogen ions then diffuse into the tubular urine, where they displace basic ions (most often sodium) from a basic salt of a weak acid and thereby change the basic salt to an acid salt or to a weak acid that is eliminated in the urine. While this is happening, the displaced sodium or other basic ion diffuses into a tubule cell. Here, it combines with the bicarbonate ion left over from the carbonic acid dissociation to form sodium bicarbonate. The sodium bicarbonate then diffuses—is reabsorbed—into the blood. Consider the various results of this mechanism. Sodium bicarbonate (or other basic bicarbonate) is conserved for the body. Instead of all the basic salts that filter out of glomerular blood, leaving the body in the urine, considerable amounts are recovered into peritubular capillary blood. In addition, extra hydrogen ions are added to the urine and thereby eliminated from the body. Both the reabsorption of base bicarbonate into blood and the excretion of hydrogen ions into urine tend to increase the ratio of the bicarbonate buffer pair $B \cdot HCO_3/H \cdot HCO_3$ (BB/CA) present in blood. This automatically increases blood pH. In short, kidney tubule base bicarbonate reabsorption and hydrogen ion excretion both tend to alkalinize blood by acidifying urine.

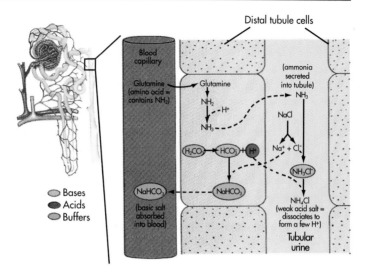

Acidification of urine by tubule excretion of ammonia (NH₃). An amino acid (glutamine) moves into the tubule cell and loses an amino group (NH₂) to form ammonia, which is secreted into urine. In exchange, the tubule cell reabsorbs a basic salt (mainly NaHCO₃) into blood from urine. Renal tubule excretion of hydrogen and ammonia is controlled at least in part by the blood pH level. A decrease in blood pH accelerates tubule excretion of both hydrogen and ammonia. An increase in blood pH produces the opposite effects.

$\mathscr{A}$cid–Base Imbalances

All of the buffer pairs in body fluids play an important role in acid-base balance. However, only in the bicarbonate system can the body regulate quickly and precisely the levels of both chemical components in the buffer pair. Carbonic acid levels can be regulated by the respiratory system and bicarbonate ion by the kidneys. A 20:1 ratio of base bicarbonate to carbonic acid (BB:CA) will, according to the Henderson-Hasselbalch equation, maintain acid-base balance and normal blood pH. Therefore, from a clinical standpoint, disturbances in acid-base balance depend on the relative quantities of carbonic acid and base bicarbonate in the extracellular fluid. Two types of disturbances, metabolic and respiratory, can alter the proper ratio of these components. Metabolic disturbances affect the bicarbonate element, and respiratory disturbances affect the carbonic acid element of the buffer pair.

Metabolic and respiratory acidosis, for example, are separate and very different types of acid-base imbalances. Both are treated by the intravenous infusion of solutions containing sodium lactate. The infused lactate ions are metabolized by liver cells and converted to bicarbonate ions. This therapy helps replace the depleted bicarbonate reserves required to restore acid-base balance in metabolic acidosis. In respiratory acidosis the additional bicarbonate ions function to offset elevated carbonic acid levels.

*M*etabolic Disturbances

METABOLIC ACIDOSIS (BICARBONATE DEFICIT)

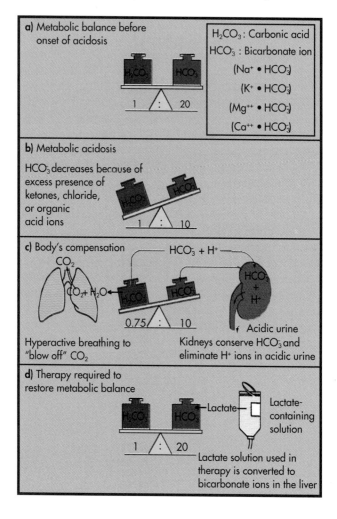

a) Metabolic balance before onset of acidosis

H_2CO_3 : Carbonic acid
HCO_3^- : Bicarbonate ion
$(Na^+ \cdot HCO_3^-)$
$(K^+ \cdot HCO_3^-)$
$(Mg^{++} \cdot HCO_3^-)$
$(Ca^{++} \cdot HCO_3^-)$

H_2CO_3 HCO_3
1 : 20

b) Metabolic acidosis

HCO_3 decreases because of excess presence of ketones, chloride, or organic acid ions

H_2CO_3 HCO_3
1 : 10

c) Body's compensation

CO_2
$CO_2 + H_2O$

$HCO_3^- + H^+$

H_2CO_3 HCO_3
0.75 : 10

HCO_3^-
+
H^+

Acidic urine

Hyperactive breathing to "blow off" CO_2

Kidneys conserve HCO_3 and eliminate H^+ ions in acidic urine

d) Therapy required to restore metabolic balance

H_2CO_3 HCO_3 — Lactate

Lactate-containing solution

1 : 20

Lactate solution used in therapy is converted to bicarbonate ions in the liver

During the course of certain diseases such as untreated diabetes mellitus, or during starvation, abnormally large amounts of acids enter the blood. The ratio of BB:CA is altered as the base bicarbonate component of the buffer pair reacts with the acids. The result may be a new ratio near 10:1. The decreasing ratio lowers the blood pH, and the respiratory center is stimulated. The resulting hyperventilation results in a "blow-off" of carbon dioxide, with a decrease in carbonic acid. This compensatory action of the respiratory system, coupled with excretion of H^+ and NH_3 in exchange for reabsorbed Na^+ by the kidneys, may be sufficient to adjust the *ratio* of BB:CA, and therefore blood pH, to normal. (The compensated BB:CA ratio may approach 10:0.5.) If, despite these compensating homeostatic devices, the ratio and pH cannot be corrected, uncompensated metabolic acidosis develops.

Increased blood hydrogen ion concentration, that is, decreased blood pH, stimulates the respiratory center. For this reason, hyperventilation is an outstanding clinical sign of acidosis. Increases in hydrogen ion concentration above a certain level depress the central nervous system and therefore produce such symptoms as disorientation and coma. In a terminal illness, death from acidosis is likely to follow coma, whereas death from alkalosis generally follows tetany and convulsions.

METABOLIC ALKALOSIS (BICARBONATE EXCESS)

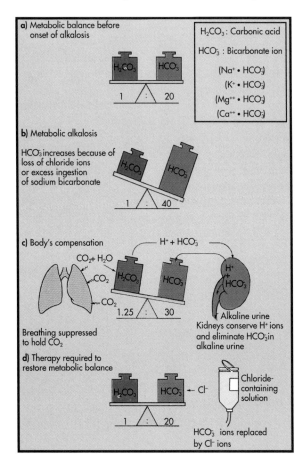

Patients suffering from chronic stomach problems such as hyper-acidity sometimes ingest large quantities of alkali—often the alkali is plain baking soda, or may be simply sodium bicarbonate for extended periods of time. Such improper use of antacids or excessive vomiting can produce metabolic alkalosis. Initially the condition results in an increase in the BB:CA ratio to perhaps 40:1. Compensatory mechanisms are aimed at increasing carbonic acid levels and decreasing the bicarbonate load. With breathing suppressed and the kidneys excreting bicarbonate ions, a compensated ratio of 30:1.24 might result. Such a ratio would restore acid-base balance and blood pH to normal. In uncompensated metabolic alkalosis the ratio, and therefore the pH, remain increased.

$\mathscr{R}$espiratory Disturbances

RESPIRATORY ACIDOSIS (CARBONIC ACID EXCESS)

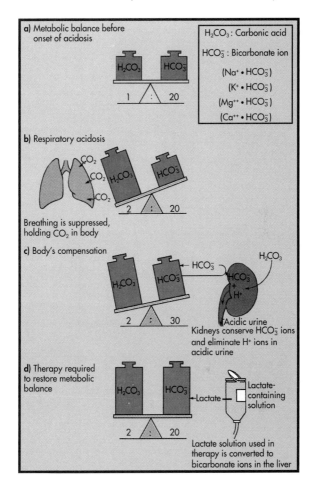

a) Metabolic balance before onset of acidosis

H_2CO_3 : Carbonic acid
HCO_3^- : Bicarbonate ion
$(Na^+ \cdot HCO_3^-)$
$(K^+ \cdot HCO_3^-)$
$(Mg^{++} \cdot HCO_3^-)$
$(Ca^{++} \cdot HCO_3^-)$

H_2CO_3 HCO_3^-

1 : 20

b) Respiratory acidosis

CO_2
CO_2 H_2CO_3 HCO_3^-
CO_2

2 : 20

Breathing is suppressed, holding CO_2 in body

c) Body's compensation

H_2CO_3 HCO_3^- $\leftarrow HCO_3^-$ H_2CO_3
HCO_3^-
+
H^+

2 : 30

Acidic urine
Kidneys conserve HCO_3^- ions and eliminate H^+ ions in acidic urine

d) Therapy required to restore metabolic balance

H_2CO_3 HCO_3^- $\leftarrow$ Lactate
Lactate-containing solution

2 : 20

Lactate solution used in therapy is converted to bicarbonate ions in the liver

Clinical conditions such as pneumonia or emphysema tend to cause retention of carbon dioxide in the blood. Also, drug abuse or overdose, such as barbiturate poisoning, will suppress breathing and result in respiratory acidosis. The carbonic acid component of the bicarbonate buffer pair increases above normal in respiratory acidosis. Body compensation, if successful, increases the bicarbonate fraction so that a new BB:CA ratio (perhaps 20:2) will return blood pH to normal or near normal levels.

RESPIRATORY ALKALOSIS (CARBONIC ACID DEFICIT)

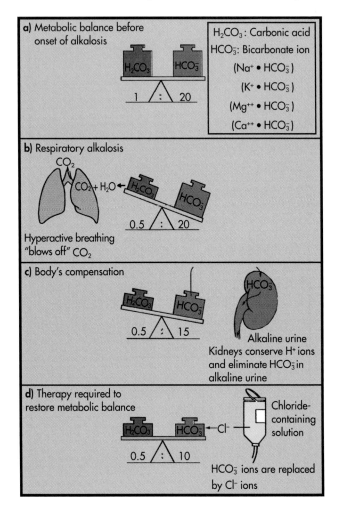

a) Metabolic balance before onset of alkalosis

H_2CO_3 HCO_3^-

1 : 20

H_2CO_3: Carbonic acid
HCO_3^-: Bicarbonate ion
$(Na^+ \bullet HCO_3^-)$
$(K^+ \bullet HCO_3^-)$
$(Mg^{++} \bullet HCO_3^-)$
$(Ca^{++} \bullet HCO_3^-)$

b) Respiratory alkalosis

CO_2

$CO_2 + H_2O \leftarrow H_2CO_3$ HCO_3^-

0.5 : 20

Hyperactive breathing "blows off" CO_2

c) Body's compensation

H_2CO_3 HCO_3^-

0.5 : 15

HCO_3^-

Alkaline urine
Kidneys conserve H^+ ions and eliminate HCO_3^- in alkaline urine

d) Therapy required to restore metabolic balance

H_2CO_3 HCO_3^- ← Cl^-

0.5 : 10

Chloride-containing solution

HCO_3^- ions are replaced by Cl^- ions

Hyperventilation caused by fever or mental disease (hysteria) can result in excessive loss of carbonic acid and lead to respiratory alkalosis with a bicarbonate buffer pair ratio of 20:0.5. Compensatory mechanisms may adjust the ratio to 10:0.5 and return blood pH to near normal.

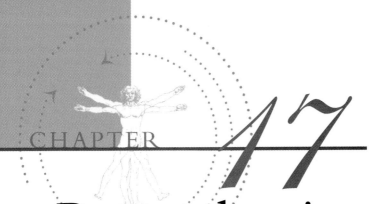

Reproductive Systems

In both sexes, organs of the reproductive system are adapted for the specific sequence of functions that are concerned primarily with propagation of the species. Production of hormones that permit the development of secondary sex characteristics occurs as a result of normal reproductive activity.

*M*ale Reproductive Organs

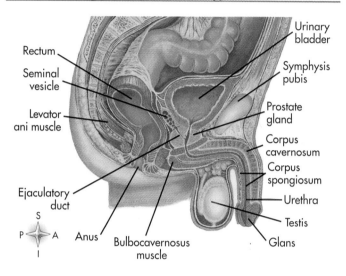

Sagittal section of the pelvis showing placement of male reproductive organs.

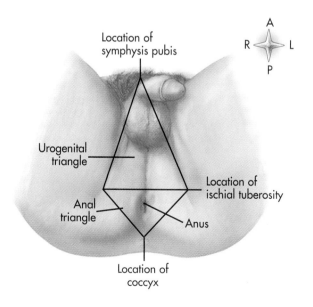

Male perineum showing outline of the urogenital and anal triangles.

$\mathscr{S}$eminiferous Tubule

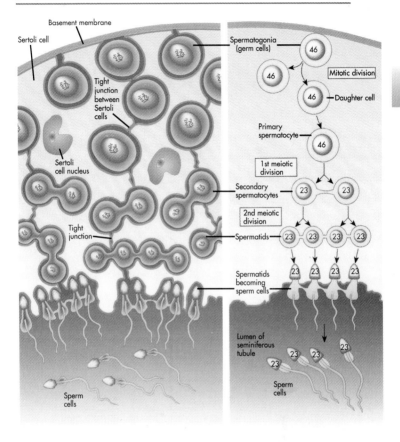

Section showing the process of meiosis and sperm formation.

*D*evelopment of Sperm

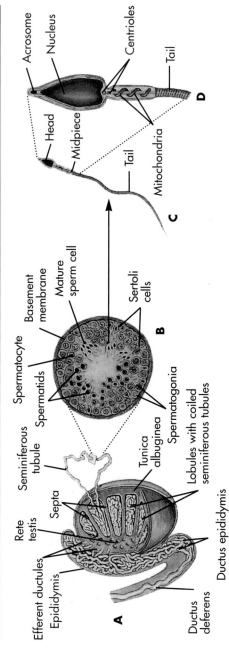

A, View of the testis and seminiferous tubules. **B,** Spermatid cells. **C,** Mature sperm. **D,** Enlarged view of the head and midpiece of the sperm.

$\mathscr{T}$he Male Reproductive System

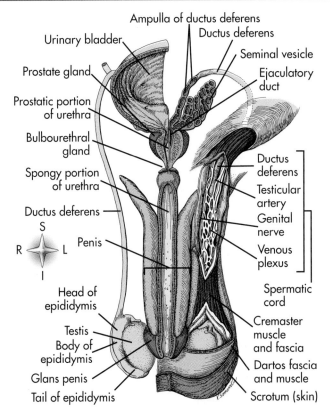

Ampulla of ductus deferens
Ductus deferens
Urinary bladder
Prostate gland
Seminal vesicle
Ejaculatory duct
Prostatic portion of urethra
Bulbourethral gland
Spongy portion of urethra
Ductus deferens
Testicular artery
Genital nerve
Venous plexus
Penis
Spermatic cord
Head of epididymis
Cremaster muscle and fascia
Testis
Body of epididymis
Dartos fascia and muscle
Glans penis
Tail of epididymis
Scrotum (skin)

This illustration shows the testes, epididymis, ductus deferens, and glands of the male reproductive system in an isolation/dissection format.

$\mathscr{F}$emale Pelvic Organs

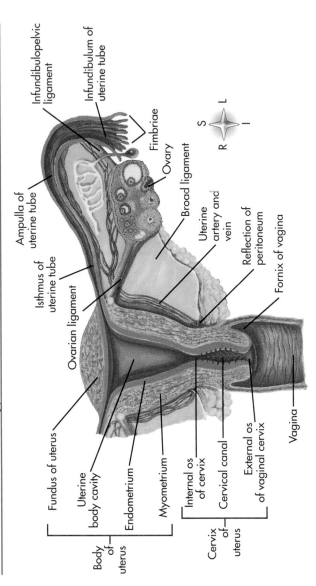

The entire uterus is shown in this frontal section of the female pelvic organs, including the upper portion of the vagina and the left uterine tube and ovary.

Female Reproductive System

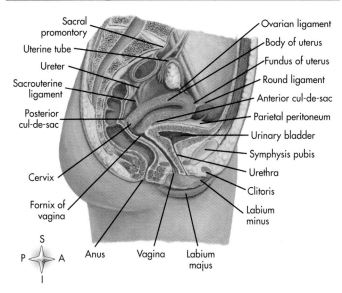

Sacral promontory
Uterine tube
Ureter
Sacrouterine ligament
Posterior cul-de-sac
Cervix
Fornix of vagina

Ovarian ligament
Body of uterus
Fundus of uterus
Round ligament
Anterior cul-de-sac
Parietal peritoneum
Urinary bladder
Symphysis pubis
Urethra
Clitoris
Labium minus

S
P — A
I

Anus   Vagina   Labium majus

Sagittal section of the pelvis shows the location of female reproductive organs.

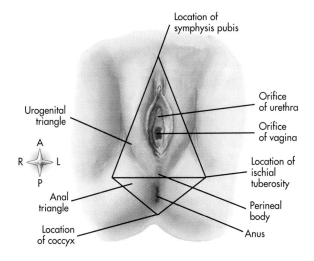

Location of symphysis pubis

Urogenital triangle

A
R — L
P

Anal triangle

Location of coccyx

Orifice of urethra
Orifice of vagina
Location of ischial tuberosity
Perineal body
Anus

The female perineum showing the outline of the urogenital and anal triangles. (Pubic hair has been removed to show detail).

*S*tages of Ovarian Follicle Development

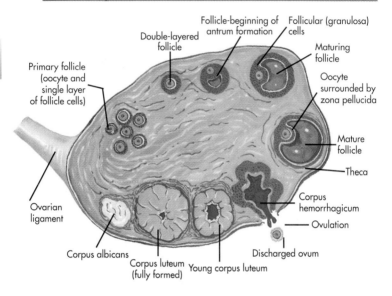

This artist's depiction shows the successive stages of ovarian follicle and oocyte development. Begin with the first stage (primary follicle) and follow around clockwise to the final stage (corpus albicans). Remember, however, that all the stages shown occur over time to a *single* follicle, and the presence of all these stages at a single point in time is an artificial construct for learning purposes only.

External Genitals of the Female

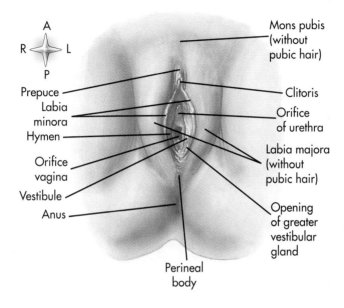

The external genitals of the female, together, constitute the external genitals, or vulva. Coarse pubic hairs appear on the mons pubis at puberty and persist throughout life. (No pubic hair is shown on this illustration.)

𝒯he Female Breast

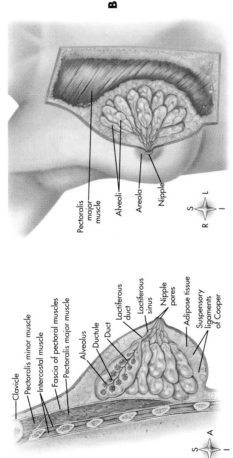

Labels in figure A: Clavicle, Pectoralis minor muscle, Intercostal muscle, Fascia of pectoral muscles, Pectoralis major muscle, Alveolus, Ductule, Duct, Lactiferous duct, Lactiferous sinus, Nipple pores, Adipose tissue, Suspensory ligaments of Cooper

Labels in figure B: Pectoralis major muscle, Alveoli, Areola, Nipple

A, Sagittal section of a lactating breast. Notice how the glandular structures are anchored to the overlying skin and to the pectoral muscles by the suspensory ligaments of Cooper. Each lobule of glandular tissue is drained by a lactiferous duct that eventually opens through the nipple. **B,** Anterior view of a lactating breast. Overlying skin and connective tissue have been removed from the medial side to show the internal structure of the breast and underlying skeletal muscle. In nonlactating breasts, the glandular tissue is much less prominent, with adipose tissue comprising most of each breast.

*L*actation

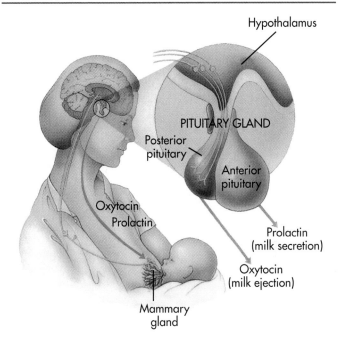

This illustration summarizes the mechanisms that control the secretion and ejection of milk.

The Primary Effects of Gonadotropins on the Ovaries

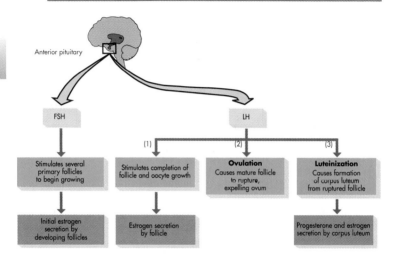

Follicle-stimulating hormone *(FSH)* gets its name from the fact that it triggers the development of primary ovarian follicles and stimulates follicular cells to secrete estrogens. Luteinizing hormone *(LH)* has several effects on ovaries: (1) LH acts as synergist to FSH to enhance its effects on follicular development and secretion; (2) LH presumably triggers ovulation—hence it is called "the ovulating hormone"; and (3) there is a luteinizing effect of LH (for which the hormone was named); recent evidence shows that FSH is also necessary for luteinization.

Female Reproductive Cycles

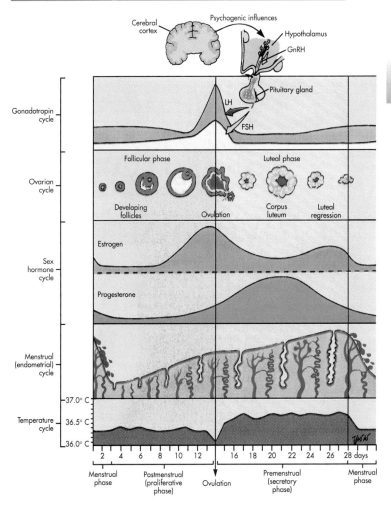

This diagram illustrates the interrelationships among the cerebral, hypothalamic, pituitary, ovarian, and uterine functions throughout a standard 28-day menstrual cycle. The variations in basal body temperature are also illustrated here.

18

Growth, Development, and Genetics

Before a new human life can begin, some preliminary processes must occur. Of utmost importance is the production of mature *gametes,* or sex cells, by each parent. Spermatozoa, gametes of the male parent, are produced by a process called *spermatogenesis.* Ova, gametes of the female parent, are produced by a process called *oogenesis.*

*M*eiotic Cell Division

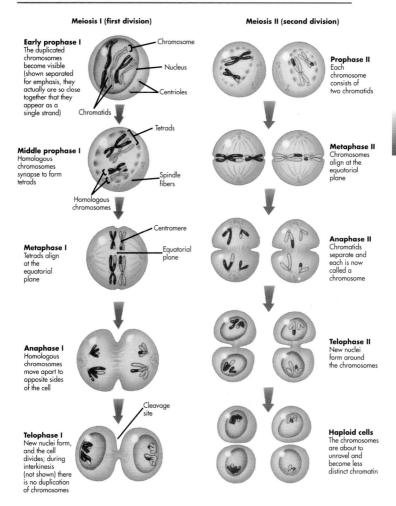

Meiosis I (first division)

Early prophase I
The duplicated chromosomes become visible (shown separated for emphasis, they actually are so close together that they appear as a single strand)

Chromosome

Nucleus

Centrioles

Chromatids

Middle prophase I
Homologous chromosomes synapse to form tetrads

Tetrads

Spindle fibers

Homologous chromosomes

Metaphase I
Tetrads align at the equatorial plane

Centromere

Equatorial plane

Anaphase I
Homologous chromosomes move apart to opposite sides of the cell

Telophase I
New nuclei form, and the cell divides; during interkinesis (not shown) there is no duplication of chromosomes

Cleavage site

Meiosis II (second division)

Prophase II
Each chromosome consists of two chromatids

Metaphase II
Chromosomes align at the equatorial plane

Anaphase II
Chromatids separate and each is now called a chromosome

Telophase II
New nuclei form around the chromosomes

Haploid cells
The chromosomes are about to unravel and become less distinct chromatin

Meiosis occurs in a series of two divisions called meiosis I and meiosis II. Notice in the illustration above that four daughter cells, each with the haploid number of chromosomes, are produced from each parent cell that enters meiotic cell division. For simplicity's sake, only four chromosomes are shown in the parent cell instead of the usual 46.

*O*ogenesis

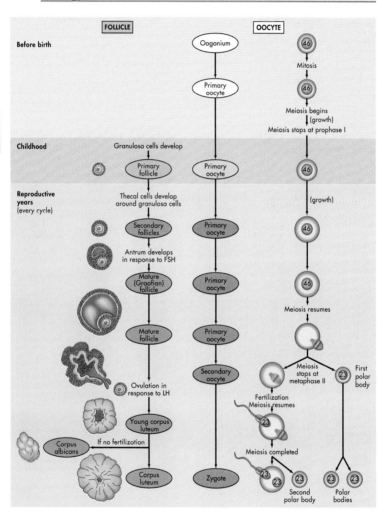

Production of a mature ovum (oocyte) and subsequent fertilization are shown *on the right* as a series of cell divisions and *on the left* as a series of changes in the ovarian follicle.

Fertilization and Implantation

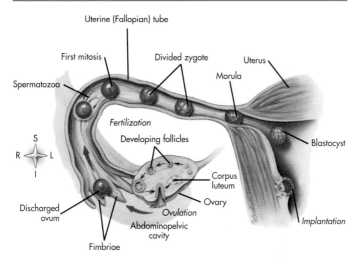

At ovulation, an ovum is released from the ovary and begins its journey through the uterine tube. While in the tube, the ovum unites with a sperm to form the single-celled zygote. After a few days of rapid mitotic division, a ball of cells called a *morula* is formed. After the morula develops into a hollow ball called a *blastocyst*, implantation occurs.

*F*ertilization to Implantation and Development of the Yolk Sac

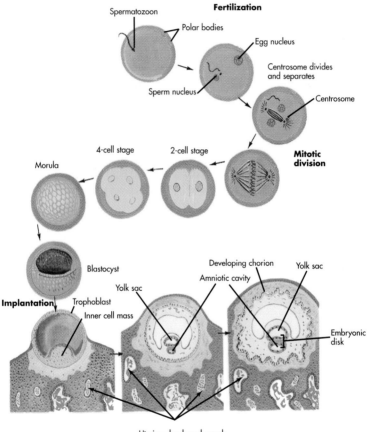

Fertilization

Spermatozoon
Polar bodies
Egg nucleus
Sperm nucleus
Centrosome divides and separates
Centrosome
Mitotic division
2-cell stage
4-cell stage
Morula
Implantation
Blastocyst
Trophoblast
Inner cell mass
Yolk sac
Developing chorion
Amniotic cavity
Yolk sac
Embryonic disk
Uterine glands and vessels

Rapid growth of uterine glands and vessels covers the developing blastocyst at the time of implantation.

$\mathscr{D}$evelopment of the Chorion and Amnion

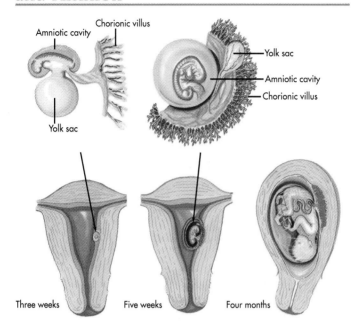

The illustration shows the development of the chorion and amniotic cavity up to 4 months of gestation.

*S*tructural Features of the Placenta

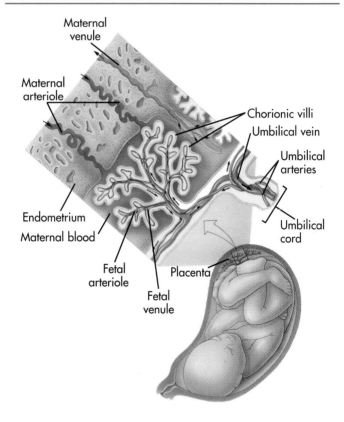

Maternal venule

Maternal arteriole

Chorionic villi

Umbilical vein

Umbilical arteries

Endometrium

Maternal blood

Umbilical cord

Fetal arteriole

Placenta

Fetal venule

The close placement of the fetal blood supply and maternal blood supply permits diffusion of nutrients and other substances. It also forms a thin barrier to prevent diffusion of most harmful substances. No mixing of fetal and maternal blood occurs.

$\mathscr{H}$ormone Levels During Pregnancy

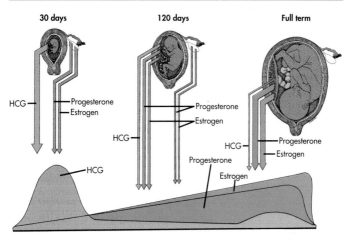

This diagram shows the changes that occur in the blood concentration of human chorionic gonadotropin (HCG), estrogen, and progesterone during gestation. Note that high HCG levels produced by placental tissue early in pregnancy maintain estrogen and progesterone secretion by the corpus luteum. This prevents menstruation and promotes maintenance of the uterine lining. As the placenta takes over the job of secreting estrogen and progesterone, HCG levels drop, and the corpus luteum subsequently ceases secreting these hormones.

$\mathcal{N}$ormal Intrauterine Fetal Position in Full-Term Pregnancy

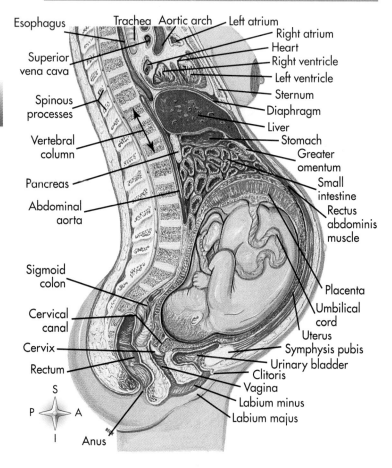

Esophagus — Trachea — Aortic arch — Left atrium

Right atrium
Heart
Right ventricle
Left ventricle
Sternum
Diaphragm
Liver
Stomach
Greater omentum
Small intestine
Rectus abdominis muscle

Superior vena cava

Spinous processes

Vertebral column

Pancreas

Abdominal aorta

Sigmoid colon

Cervical canal

Cervix

Rectum

Placenta
Umbilical cord
Uterus
Symphysis pubis
Urinary bladder
Clitoris
Vagina
Labium minus
Labium majus

S
P — A
I

Anus

This illustration shows the normal intrauterine position of a fetus just before birth in a full-term pregnancy.

Human Chromosomes

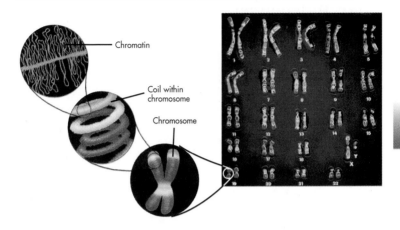

Chromatin

Coil within
chromosome

Chromosome

Each of the 46 human chromosomes, arranged here in numbered pairs for easy reference, is a coiled mass of chromatin (DNA). In this figure, differentially stained bands in each chromosome appear as different bright colors. Such bands are useful as reference points when identifying the locations of specific genes within a chromosome. (© Photo Researchers, Inc.)

*M*eiosis and the Principle of Independent Assortment

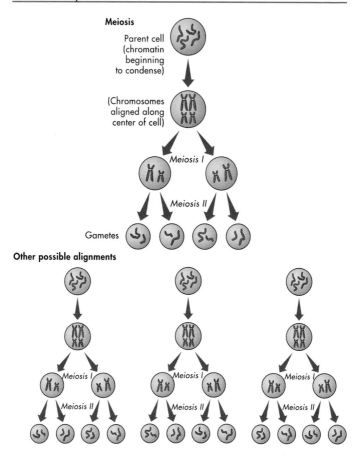

In meiosis, a series of two divisions results in the production of gametes with half the number of chromosomes of the original parent cell. In both meiotic divisions shown here, the original cell has four chromosomes and gametes each have two chromosomes. During the first division of meiosis, pairs of similar chromosomes line up along the cell's equator for even distribution to daughter cells. Because different pairs assort independently of each other, four (2^2) different alignments of chromosomes can occur. Because human cells have 23 pairs of chromosomes, over 8 million (2^{23}) different combinations are possible.

Crossing Over

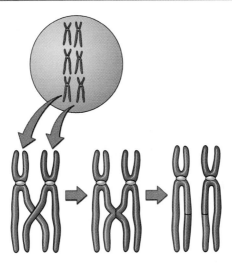

Genes (or linked groups of genes) from one chromosome are exchanged with matching genes in the other chromosome of a pair during meiosis.

Inheritance of Albinism

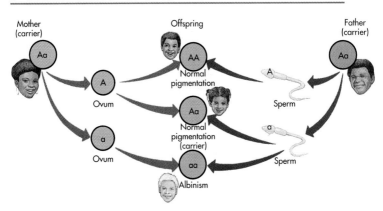

Albinism is an example of a recessive trait, producing abnormalities only in those with two recessive genes *(a)*. Presence of the dominant gene *(A)* prevents albinism.

*S*ex Determination

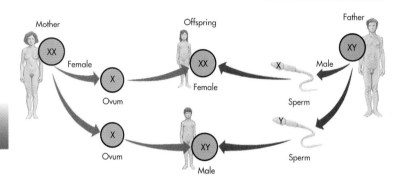

The presence of the Y chromosome specifies maleness. In the absence of a Y chromosome, an individual develops into a female.

*S*ex-Linked Inheritance

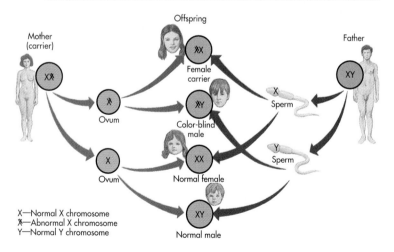

X—Normal X chromosome
X̶—Abnormal X chromosome
Y—Normal Y chromosome

Some forms of color blindness involve recessive X-linked genes. In the illustration, a female carrier of the abnormal gene can produce male children who are color blind.

Effects of Nondisjunction

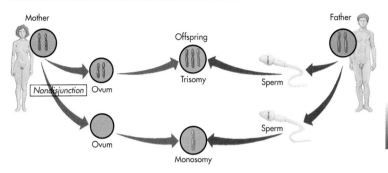

Nondisjunction, failure of a chromosome pair to separate during gamete production, may result in trisomy or monosomy in the offspring.

Examples of Genetic Conditions

Chromosome Location	Disease	Description
Single-Gene Inheritance (Nuclear DNA)		
Dominant		
7, 17	Osteogenesis imperfecta	Group of connective tissue disorders is characterized by imperfect skeletal development that produces brittle bones
17	Multiple neurofibromatosis	Disorder is characterized by multiple, sometimes disfiguring benign tumors of the Schwann cells (neuroglia) that surround nerve fibers
5	Hypercholesterolemia	High blood cholesterol may lead to atherosclerosis and other cardiovascular problems
4	Huntington disease (HD)	Degenerative brain disorder is characterized by chorea (purposeless movements) progressing to severe dementia and death generally by age 55
Codominant		
11	Sickle-cell anemia Sickle-cell trait	Blood disorder in which abnormal hemoglobin causes red blood cells (RBCs) to deform into a sickle shape; sickle-cell anemia is the severe form, and sickle-cell trait the milder form
11, 16	Thalassemia	Group of inherited hemoglobin disorders is characterized by production of hypochromic, abnormal RBCs
Recessive (autosomal)		
7	Cystic fibrosis (CF)	Condition is characterized by excessive secretion of thick mucus and concentrated sweat, often causing obstruction of gastrointestinal or respiratory ducts
15	Tay-Sachs disease	Fatal condition in which abnormal lipids accumulate in the brain and cause tissue damage leading to death by age 4
12	Phenylketonuria (PKU)	Excess of phenylketones in the urine is caused by accumulation of phenylalanine in the tissues; it may cause brain injury and death if phenylalanine (amino acid) intake is not managed properly

11	Albinism (total)	Lack of the dark brown pigment *melanin* in the skin and eyes results in vision problems and susceptibility to sunburn and skin cancer
20	Severe combined immune deficiency (SCID)	Failure of the lymphocytes to develop properly causes failure of the immune system's defense of the body; it is usually caused by adenosine deaminase (ADA) deficiency
Recessive (X-linked)		
23 (X)	Hemophilia	Group of blood clotting disorders is caused by failure to form clotting factors VIII, IX, or XI
23 (X)	Duchenne muscular dystrophy (DMD)	Muscle disorder is characterized by progressive atrophy of skeletal muscle without nerve involvement
23 (X)	Red-green color blindness	Inability to distinguish red and green light results from a deficiency of photopigments in the cone cells of the retina
23 (X)	Fragile X syndrome	Mental retardation results from breakage of X chromosome in males
23 (X)	Ocular albinism	Form of albinism in which the pigmented layers of the eyeball lack melanin; results in hypersensitivity to light and other problems
23 (X)	Androgen insensitivity	Inherited insensitivity to androgens (steroid sex hormones associated with maleness) results in reduced effects of these hormones
23 (X)	Cleft palate (X-linked form)	One form of a congenital deformity in which the skull fails to develop properly; it is characterized by a gap in the palate (plate separating mouth from nasal cavity)
23 (X)	Retinitis pigmentosa	Condition causes blindness, characterized by clumps of melanin in retina of eyes
SINGLE-GENE INHERITANCE (MITOCHONDRIAL DNA)		
mDNA	Leber hereditary optic neuropathy	Optic nerve degeneration in young adults results in total blindness by age 30
mDNA	Parkinson disease (?)	Nervous disorder is characterized by involuntary trembling and muscle rigidity

$\mathscr{P}$edigree

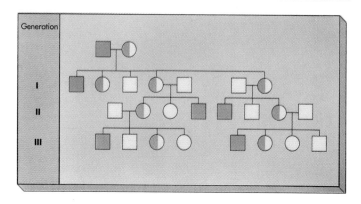

Pedigrees chart the genetic history of family lines. *Squares* represent males, and circles represent females. Fully shaded symbols indicate affected individuals, *partly shaded symbols* indicate carriers, and *unshaded symbols* indicate unaffected noncarriers. *Roman numerals* indicate the order of generations. This particular pedigree reveals the presence of an X-linked recessive trait.

Punnett Square

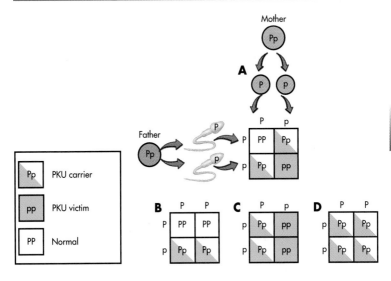

The Punnett square is a grid used to determine relative probabilities of producing offspring with specific gene combinations. Phenylketonuria (PKU) is a recessive disorder caused by the gene *p*. *P* is the normal gene. **A,** Possible results of cross between two PKU carriers. Because one in four of the offspring represented in the grid have PKU, a genetic counselor would predict a 25% chance that this couple will produce a PKU baby at each birth. **B,** Cross between a PKU carrier and a normal noncarrier. **C,** Cross between a PKU victim and a PKU carrier. **D,** Cross between a PKU victim and a normal noncarrier.

$\mathscr{P}$hoto and Illustration Credits

AP Wide World Photos, New York, New York.
Edward L. Applebaum, University of Illinois.
Peter Arnold Inc., New York, New York.
Lester V. Bergman & Associates, Cold Spring, New York.
Berne RM, Levy MN: *Cardiovascular physiology,* ed. 6, St Louis, 1992, Mosby.
Bevelander G, Ramaley JA: *Essentials of histology,* ed. 8, St Louis, 1978, Mosby.
Biological Photo Services, Moss Beach, California.
Robert L. Calentine, River Falls, Wisconsin.
Custom Medical Stock Photo, Chicago, Illinois.
Daffner RH: *Introduction to clinical radiation,* St Louis, 1978, Mosby.
Ron Edwards, Chesterfield, Missouri.
Erlandsen SL, Magney J: *Color atlas of histology,* St Louis, 1992, Mosby.
Andrew P. Evan, Indiana University.
Charles Flickinger, University of Virginia.
Fujita T, Tanaka K, Tokunaga J, editors: *SEM atlas of cells and tissues,* Tokyo, Japan, 1981, Igaku-Shoin Publishers.
James A. Ischen, Baylor College of Medicine, Houston, Texas.
Ishihara: *Tests for colour blindness,* Tokyo, Japan, 1973, Kanehara Shuppan Co. Ltd.
Susumu Ito, Harvard Medical School.
Lanny L. Johnson, MD, East Lansing, Michigan.
Patricia Kane, Indiana University Medical School.
Kessel RG, Kardon RH: *Tissues and organs: a text atlas of scanning electron microscopy,* 1979, WH Freeman.
Loris McGavran, Denver Children's Hospital.
Scott Mittman, MD, Johns Hopkins Hospital, Baltimore, Maryland.
Lennart Nilsson, Albert Bonniers Forlag AB, Stockholm, Sweden.
Nolte J, Angevine JB Jr: *The human brain in photographs and diagrams,* St Louis, 1995, Mosby.
MM Perry, Edinburgh Research Center.
Photo Researchers, Inc., New York, New York.
Phototake, New York, New York.
Potter PA, Perry AG: *Fundamentals of nursing: concepts, process, and practice,* ed. 4, St Louis, 1997, Mosby.
Ed Reschke, Muskegon, Michigan.
Brenda Russell, PhD, University of Illinois at Chicago, Chicago, Illinois.
Seidel et al: *Mosby's guide to physical examination,* ed. 4, St Louis, 1999, Mosby.
Simon C, Janner M: *Color atlas of pediatric diseases,* ed. 4, 1988, Chapman & Hall, ITP International Thomson Publishing.
Stewart Halperin Photography, St Louis, Missouri.
Ivan Stotz, South Dakota State University.
Walter Tunnessen, MD, The American Board of Pediatrics, Chapel Hill, North Carolina.
Veeck L: *Atlas of the human oocyte and early conceptus,* vol 1, 1986, Baltimore, Williams & Wilkins.
Visuals Unlimited, Inc., Swanzey, New Hampshire.
Nancy Wexler, Columbia University.

Index

A

A band, *178*
Abdomen
  division of, into four
    quadrants, *10*
  transverse section of,
    464
Abdominal aorta, de-
  scending, 379t-
  380t
Abdominal cavity, organs
  in, 5t
Abdominal wall, muscles
  of, 190t, 197t-
  198t, *199*
Abdominopelvic cavity,
  organs in, 5t
Abdominopelvic cavity,
  regions of, *9-10*
Abducens nerve, 290t
Abduction, joint move-
  ments and, 173t
Abductor digiti minimi
  muscle, 213t, 229t
Abductor hallucis muscle,
  229t
Abductor pollicis brevis
  muscle, 212t
Absorption, 464t
Absorption sites in
  digestive tract,
  481
Accessory nerve, 294t
Acetabulum, 150t
Acetoacetate, urinalysis
  and, 517t
Acetone, urinalysis and,
  517t
Acetylcholine (ACh), 181,
  246, 248t, *303*
Acetyl-CoA, *490*
ACh; *see* Acetylcholine

Acid phosphatase, blood
  values and, 355t
Acid secretion by gastric
  parietal cells, *472*
Acid-base balance, fluids
  and electrolytes
  and, 520-544
Acid-base imbalances,
  539
Acquired immunity, 419t
Acromioclavicular joint,
  170t
Acromion process, 138t
Action potential, *243*,
  244t
Active transport, 51t, 58,
  478
Adduction, joint
  movements and,
  173t
Adductor group muscles,
  219t
Adductor pollicis muscle,
  212t
Adductor tubercle, 152t
Adenine, 37
Adenohypophysis, *337*,
  338
Adenosine diphosphate
  (ADP), 38, *183*,
  488
Adenosine triphosphate
  (ATP), 38, *59*,
  181, *247*, 483-
  484, *489*
ADH; *see* Antidiuretic
  hormone
Adipose tissue, *90*
ADP; *see* Adenosine
  diphosphate
Adrenal androgens, 344t
Adrenal estrogens, 344t

Adrenal glands, 329t
  hormones of, 344t
  structure of, *343*
Adrenaline, 344t
Aerobic pathway, *486*
Afferent arteriole, *507*
Air sinuses, 127t
Albinism, 573t
  inheritance of, *569*
  ocular, 573t
Albumin
  blood values and, 360t
  membrane permeable
    to, *54*
  urinalysis and, 517t
Aldosterone, *332, 343*,
  344t, *397, 526*
Alkali, *542*
Alkaline phosphatase,
  blood values and,
  355t
Allosteric effect, *62*
Alveolar process, 125t
Alveolus, *427*
Amines, 248t
Amino acid derivatives,
  331, 333
Amino acids, 249t, 492t
  absorption of, *478*
  basic structural formula
    for, *25*
Ammonia, 517t, 538
Amnion, development of,
  563
Amniotic cavity, *563*
Amphiarthrotic joints,
  170t-172t
Amylase, 470t
Anaerobic pathway, *486*
Anal triangle
  female, *551*
  male, *546*

Italic page numbers indicate illustrations; page numbers followed by t indicate tables.

Word Parts Commonly Used as Prefixes

WORD PART	MEANING
a-	Without, not
af-	Toward
an-	Without, not
ante-	Before
anti-	Against; resisting
auto-	Self
bi-	Two; double
circum-	Around
co-, con-	With; together
contra-	Against
de-	Down from, undoing
dia-	Across, through
dipl-	Twofold, double
dys-	Bad; disordered; difficult
ectop-	Displaced
ef-	Away from
em-, en-	In, into
endo-	Within
epi-	Upon
eu-	Good
ex-, exo-	Out of, out from
extra-	Outside of
hapl-	Single
hem-, hemat-	Blood
hemi-	Half
hom(e)o-	Same; equal
hyper-	Over; above
hypo-	Under; below
infra-	Below; beneath
inter-	Between
intra-	Within
iso-	Same, equal
macro-	Large
mega-	Large; million(th)
mes-	Middle
meta-	Beyond, after
micro-	Small; millionth
milli-	Thousandth
mono-	One (single)
neo-	New
non-	Not
oligo-	Few, scanty
ortho-	Straight; correct, normal
para-	By the side of; near
per-	Through
peri-	Around; surrounding
poly-	Many
post-	After
pre-	Before
pro-	First; promoting
quadr-	Four
re-	Back again
retro-	Behind
semi-	Half
sub-	Under
super-, supra-	Over, above, excessive
trans-	Across; through
tri-	Three; triple

Word Parts Commonly Used as Suffixes

WORD PART	MEANING
-al, -ac	Pertaining to
-algia	Pain
-aps, -apt	Fit; fasten
-arche	Beginning; origin
-ase	Signifies an enzyme
-blast	Sprout; make
-centesis	A piercing
-cide	To kill
-clast	Break; destroy
-crine	Release; secrete
-ectomy	A cutting out
-emesis	Vomiting
-emia	Refers to blood condition
-flux	Flow
-gen	Creates; forms
-genesis	Creation, production
-gram	Something written
-graph(y)	To write, draw
-hydrate	Containing H_2O (water)
-ia, -sia	Condition; process
-iasis	Abnormal condition
-ic, -ac	Pertaining to
-in	Signifies a protein
-ism	Signifies "condition of"
-itis	Signifies "inflammation of"
-lemma	Rind; peel
-lepsy	Seizure
-lith	Stone; rock
-logy	Study of
-lunar	Moon; moonlike
-malacia	Softening
-megaly	Enlargement
-metric, -metry	Measurement, length
-oid	Like; in the shape of
-oma	Tumor
-opia	Vision, vision condition
-oscopy	Viewing
-ose	Signifies a carbohydrate (especially sugar)
-osis	Condition, process
-ostomy	Formation of an opening
-otomy	Cut
-penia	Lack
-philic	Loving
-phobic	Fearing
-phragm	Partition
-plasia	Growth, formation
-plasm	Substance, matter
-plasty	Shape; make
-plegia	Paralysis
-pnea	Breath, breathing
-(r)rhage, -(r)rhagia	Breaking out, discharge
-(r)rhaphy	Sew, suture
-(r)rhea	Flow
-some	Body
-tensin, -tension	Pressure
-tonic	Pressure, tension
-tripsy	Crushing
-ule	Small, little
-uria	Refers to urine condition